SMART PATIENT,
GOOD MEDICINE

SMART PATIENT, GOOD MEDICINE

Working with Your Doctor to Get the Best Medical Care

Richard L. Sribnick, M.D.,
and
Wayne B. Sribnick, M.D.

WALKER AND COMPANY
NEW YORK

First published in the United States of America in 1994
by Walker Publishing Company, Inc.

Published simultaneously in Canada by
Thomas Allen & Son Canada,
Limited, Markham, Ontario

Library of Congress Cataloging-in-Publication Data
Sribnick, Richard L.
Smart patient, good medicine : working with
your doctor to get the
best medical care / Richard L. Sribnick and Wayne B. Sribnick.
p.   cm.
Includes index.
ISBN 0-8027-1287-8. —ISBN 0-8027-7414-8 (paper)
1. Physician and patient.   2. Consumer education.   3. Patient
education   I. Sribnick, Wayne B.   II. Title.
R727.3.S75   1994
610.69'6—dc20   94-2001
CIP

Book design by Ron Monteleone

Printed in the United States of America

2   4   6   8   10   9   7   5   3

To Mom and Dad and Kevin—
without them, none of us would
have become doctors.

Contents

Acknowledgments

First, we would like to thank our patients. It is only by practicing medicine that a doctor can learn the meaning of mutual respect.

We also have a surprisingly large number of other people to thank for such a short book.

Thank you—

Linda Weingarten for your spirit and early encouragement. Jim Meriwether, Charles Pope, Vivian Marshall, Harold Marshall, Cindy McGrath, and Cliff Cleaveland for reading early drafts and offering excellent editorial advice. Ruth Butler and Sylvia Wood for hours of interviews on the patients' perspective.

Rick Silver for years of friendship and tons of advice. Mr. David Wertz for teaching us so long ago to write clearly and punctuate correctly. Alan Medlin for being as good a lawyer as he is a friend. Richard Layman for suggesting Ed Knappman, our agent, who is simply the best. Our office staff—Holly, Tranny, Lisa, Lynette, Jana, and especially, Fredia.

Our brothers and partners Dr. Michael Sribnick and Dr. Chris Durso. Lorna Durso for a sister's support and Ann Sribnick for a wife's patience and understanding.

And most of all, thank you Kathleen Marshall for more than we can possibly mention in helping to make this book a reality.

Foreword

In many of the speeches I make each year to medical consumers, I often talk about intimidation. Most of us are
intimidated by doctors. We are afraid to ask questions,
reluctant to take up too much of the physician's time, and
nervous when trying to describe our symptoms.

Our fears emanate from two sources. First is our lack
of information. We know very little about the records of
accomplishment of the doctors treating us. We have scant
knowledge about the tests, treatments, or medications
doctors order for us. Historically, there has been very little information available to consumers about matters of
medicine and health care. This lack of knowledge on our
part has made us feel meek and shy, reluctant to deal
with our medical practitioners the way we ordinarily
would interact with service providers.

Our second source of intimidation is the physician
himself (herself). Doctors do things to intimidate us. Why
do most doctors wear white coats? Nothing is going to
spill on them. They use words we do not understand.
They often do not completely listen to what we have to
say. Even the way some physicians run their offices is intimidating. For example, in many physicians' offices the
first thing a patient sees upon entering is a sign reading
"Please Make Arrangements for Payment Before Service."
A greeting like that does not engender great trust or open-
ness.

Yet despite these barriers, no consumer needs to be on

the silent end of the stethoscope. The world of medicine has changed dramatically over the last decade and it will change even more profoundly in the years to come. Each of us will be required to play a more active role in our own medical care. From choosing a physician to deciding on surgery, we must become equal partners with our health-care professionals.

This book goes a long way to help you in that process. Richard and Wayne Sribnick assist you through the process of selecting the best physician for your needs. But they do not stop there. They go on to guide you through the process of making medical decisions as an equal partner with your doctor. They break down the barriers that in the past have prevented most of us from being assertive and confident participants in our own health care.

Each year I receive tens of thousands of letters from individuals who feel short-changed by the medical system. A common lament is "If I had only known. . . ." Yet, after reading the pages that follow, written with refreshing brevity, I am confident you will become the type of empowered and informed medical consumer you have always wanted to be. And you will be surprised to find out just how unintimidating a medical encounter can be.

—Charles B. Inlander, president,
People's Medical Society

Introduction

"The doctor will see you now." The next time you hear those words, you will be calmer, more knowledgeable, and better prepared than you were during your last visit to a doctor's office.

Impossible? Not really. As a matter of fact, we are confident that a few explanations, suggestions, and guidelines will make a significant difference in your next visit with your physician. You will have a better understanding of what your doctor is doing and what you can do to help. Your participation and the effectiveness of your physician form the foundation of high quality health care. In the following chapters we discuss the diagnostic process; the components and procedures involved in patient interviews, physical exams, and testing; and the importance of identifying and choosing good doctors. We identify your role as well as your doctor's role in assuring that you receive the best possible treatment. You also will see the ways in which the roles of patient and doctor support each other.

Why is this relationship important? When you become a better and more aware patient, you enable your physician to be a more effective doctor. For too long patients have had difficulty talking to their doctors, and doctors have not emphasized how important this input is. The simple truth is that patients and doctors must learn to talk to each other. If they don't, accurate diagnoses, appropriate decisions, and patient confidence are compromised. When you and your physician approach your total health as a team, something else happens. You not only receive complete and effective care but also build a relationship of mutual trust and confidence. You feel comfortable enough to ask questions freely. The doctor is more likely to respond completely and easily to your questions. The physician may be more inclined to solicit your input and opinions when choices are possible and feel confident you will participate fully in recommended treatments.

Deciding to communicate with your doctor is no guarantee that good communication will happen. There are, however, a number of things you can do to make it happen. We are going to help you prepare for office visits, enable you to be more informed about what the doctor is doing during those examinations, and give you guidelines for asking informed and important questions. We have intentionally presented the material in a simple and concise fashion.

The first four chapters of this book are devoted to identifying and selecting a competent primary-care physician. If you already have a doctor, we show you how to assess his skills; if you don't have a doctor, we show you how to find one. When you become ill, the single most critical factor in your health care is the effectiveness of your doctor. Not only must he be competent, he must be someone you can talk to and trust. One of the descriptors we use is *primary care,* another is *specialist.* When we refer to a primary-care physician, we are talking about a doctor who focuses on the diagnosis and treatment of problems in all systems of the body. He is the doctor who will assess any type of complaint and is the one who generally gives your routine physical exam. Both the internist (practice focuses on adults) and family practitioner (practice includes adults and children) are primary-care physicians.

A specialist, on the other hand, is someone who has specialized training in one area of the body. For example, a cardiologist is a doctor who specializes in the care of the heart; a nephrologist specializes in the treatment of the kidneys.

In this section we emphasize one major point: You need to have a good primary-care physician. The quality of your health care is directly related to the quality of your doctor. You must, however, identify him first. We will give you all the information we can think of to help you do just that.

In the next section (chapters 5 through 9) we discuss the diagnostic process and its three components: the patient interview, physical examination, and diagnostic testing. You will learn how a doctor gathers information and puts it together to arrive at a conclusion. We give you the questions to ask at each step of the way.

The final four chapters continue to show how doctors and patients can work together to make effective decisions. Chapter 10 discusses the two major types of treatment: medication and surgery. Many patients want to better understand prescribed treatment but don't know what to ask. We include five questions to ask about recommended medications and five questions to ask before agreeing to surgery. Chapter 11 discusses the role of the specialist. We explore reasons why it may be necessary for you to see a specialist and provide guidelines to ensure that you receive the best care. Chapter 12 addresses doctor-patient interactions. We present five hypothetical dialogues between doctors and patients and show how each may interpret the same interaction differently. Our purpose is to promote doctor-patient understanding by illustrating each point of view. Again, in the spirit of problem solving, we conclude with a "tips" section that addresses some of the minor annoyances, such as waiting, that can

interfere needlessly with a smooth doctor-patient interaction.

Above all else, we want you to use the information provided in these pages and use it consistently. It will make
a difference—to you and your doctor.

A Note About Health-Care Delivery Systems

The health-care delivery system is constantly changing.
Fortunately, this book will enhance your knowledge and
allow you to receive the best medical care as the system
evolves. The way you pay for health care now may be different from the way you pay for health care in the future.

In all health-care delivery systems, you or your em-
ployer pay for the services provided—either directly to the
doctor, to an insurance company, or, in the case of a
single-payment government system, in the form of taxes.

In a traditional Health Maintenance Organization
(HMO), a physician is paid a set amount each year to care
for each patient, regardless of how often he sees the patient. In a Preferred Provider Organization (PPO), the
doctor is paid a predetermined fee for each visit. In traditional fee-for-service medicine, the billing is strictly between the physician and the patient; however, the patient
may be reimbursed directly by his insurance company. In
a single-payer system, the government determines the fee
and pays the physician.

The differences among these plans affect two major areas of concern to you: cost and choice. When you look at
these alternatives you may find one plan may cost less but
include fewer doctors; another may provide more services
but be more expensive. For example, in HMOs and PPOs
your choice of physicians and hospitals can only be made
from members of these organizations, but these pro-

grams may cost you less. Your decision in selecting a health-care delivery system will involve learning about each option and judging which factors are most important for your individual situation. It is possible, however, that future changes in health-care programs also may affect the range of options available to you.

With all of this in mind, you can see it is more important than ever to know how to recognize and work with a good doctor. The most important facet of high quality health care will always be the patient-doctor relationship. This is precisely what this book addresses.

SMART PATIENT, GOOD MEDICINE

1

Why You Need a Good Primary-care Doctor

Why You Need a Doctor

Have you ever thought about what you would do if you had an attack of appendicitis? What would you do if tonight you suddenly awakened with a fever and a pain in your abdomen so severe you could hardly breathe? If you have your own doctor, you would know what to do. You would call him. If, on the other hand, you didn't have a doctor, you would realize that you needed one now. In either case, you would soon be heading for the emergency room.

If you already had your own doctor, you would see someone you knew and trusted. You would feel comfortable with his ability to determine what is wrong and to recommend what's best. If you were meeting a doctor for the first time in the middle of the night you would know none of these things. Instead, you could only hope that the doctor asking you questions and examining your abdomen would do what was right. You certainly would be in no position to judge for yourself. The only thing on your mind would be how to get rid of the pain.

It is a good idea to have your own doctor. If you already have one, you need no convincing. If you don't, ask yourself: Why not? It's unlikely you would think having your own doctor is a bad idea. Rather, you've either not thought about it, don't consider it is necessary, or figure you'll get one when you need one. After all, the chances of waking up with an attack of appendicitis are rather slim. There are other reasons, however, to have your own doctor besides having someone to call in an emergency. Here are some:

1. *Having your own doctor will enable you to know the quality of care you will receive before you become ill.* The assurance of receiving high-quality care is too important to leave to chance. Even though you should participate in the decisions affecting your medical care, you need to have confidence in your physician's recommendations. There also could be life-threatening situations when you are unable to participate in the decision-making process. It's comforting to know you have a competent representative in your doctor.

2. *Your primary-care doctor can help maintain your health through consistent care and observation.* A key factor to continued good health throughout the adult years is preventive medicine and periodic examinations. If he sees you on a regular basis, a doctor is able to look for many potential problems and consistently evaluate your health. For example, high blood pressure rarely produces any symptoms but silently damages blood vessels as time goes by. The same is true of an elevated cholesterol level. There are also several common cancers (e.g., breast, prostate) that are frequently curable if detected early. Your own doctor is likely to check you periodically for problems such as these that might otherwise go undetected.

3. *Your primary-care doctor will have all your records and*

will know your medical history. One of the greatest medical advantages of having a primary-care doctor is that someone will have your medical records and know what is normal for you. This could be critical when a knowledge of previous illness or medication is important. Let's say, for example, you had three separate bladder infections in the last six months. If you had visited a walk-in clinic and seen three different doctors, it is unlikely that any of these doctors would do more than give you an antibiotic to treat the problem. If you had seen the same doctor each time, however, it would be much more likely that she would realize further testing might be needed to check for an underlying bladder abnormality.

4. *Your primary-care doctor will be able to advise you about medical or surgical procedures.* There may be occasions when another doctor recommends surgery or a specialized medical test. Your own doctor can help determine the need for surgery or intrusive medical tests and support you through the process. You can also feel more confident with the competence of the medical specialists or surgeons he recommends.

5. *Finally, your primary-care doctor is someone you can talk to easily.* You may want to discuss some personal problems you are having or ask some medical questions about an article you have read. Your own physician is more likely to be receptive to this type of conversation than a doctor you have never met. Sometimes you may need someone who will be willing to listen to you regardless of the nature of your problem. Whether it is a question about the value of calcium in your diet or a depression you are having from a recent divorce, having your own doctor allows you to seek advice from someone who already knows and cares about you as a person. The relationship between a doctor and a patient should be meaningful. It comes

from experience and time, and it provides you with a strong feeling of security when you need it most. There is no time we feel as vulnerable as when we are in pain or seriously ill.

If you haven't thought about having your own doctor before now, it's time to stop and consider its importance. Really think about getting a doctor, decide if getting one makes sense, and if you think it does—then do it.

Why Your Doctor Should Be a Good One

Because so many of the reasons you should have a primary-care doctor revolve around your trust and confidence in his abilities, it is important for you to get a *good* doctor, one who is caring and knowledgeable. This may seem self-evident or needless rhetoric, but the selection of such a doctor is a critical issue. Unless you understand why having a good doctor is so important, you might not make the effort necessary to be sure you have one.

Like it or not, things change when you get sick. You not only hurt or feel ill; you also become worried or frightened. You may have some idea why you don't feel well, but frequently you aren't certain. When you don't know the best course of action, you usually seek the opinion of someone who is more knowledgeable and skilled in dealing with the problem. A lack of knowledge and experience in areas outside our own field makes all of us feel vulnerable. When we feel this way and turn ourselves over to an expert, we are in a sense admitting our lack of information and must hope that the professional we have chosen—be it doctor, dentist, teacher, or mechanic—will do what's best. When you turn to your doctor, this vulnerability is accentuated because you almost certainly will follow his recommendations, and you realize that the consequences of his decisions can affect your future health. For example, if your doctor says you need an X-ray procedure to figure out the cause of your abdominal pain, it is likely that you will agree to have it even though you may be frightened, worried, or suspicious. You could refuse to have the test or just not show up, but it's unlikely you will do that. What if you really needed that X ray and not having it meant failing to find an ulcer in the early stage?

Whether your doctor is knowledgeable and caring or haphazard and impersonal, the doctor you choose is the one whose advice you will follow. Finding a doctor you trust is essential because it will give you the comfort of knowing his recommendations are probably the best, safest, and most effective.

Being able to trust his advice, however, is only one reason for having a good doctor rather than a less careful one. A good doctor is more likely to recommend only those tests necessary for making a diagnosis. He will base his decision for testing on knowledgeable considerations after a careful exam. This means no risks from test procedures that are not needed and less expense for you.

A skilled physician also should diagnose illnesses earlier and realize when seemingly minor symptoms represent a more significant disease. He is more likely to detect subtle findings on a physical examination and know what they represent. This doesn't mean a careful doctor never makes a mistake. Even a thorough doctor may fail to detect a small breast lump or erroneously conclude that chest pain from heart disease was indigestion. Good doesn't mean perfect. Errors in diagnosis, however, are much less likely to happen when you have a good doctor caring for you.

Doctors do more than diagnose illnesses, they also treat them. In fact, the correct choice of treatment can sometimes be more difficult than the diagnosis itself. Not only must the doctor choose the appropriate medication, he must also decide the correct dosage, consider any allergies you have, know how the drug interacts with any other medicines you take, think about possible side effects, and decide how long to treat you. That's a lot to think about. It is more likely the doctor doing the prescribing is also doing the necessary thinking if he's a good one.

The characteristics that set a good doctor apart from others include effort, judgment, caring, and concern. With an ever-expanding knowledge of disease and effective therapies, the modern doctor's ability to help his patients continues to improve. Your doctor's impact on your health can be dramatic. This fact underscores why it is so important for you to choose a highly skilled physician. As you will see in the next chapter, the process of identifying and choosing a good doctor is not necessarily easy. In this section, we hope we have convinced you that the process and the time are well worth the effort.

2

Choosing a Good Doctor

I t is surprising how little thought some people give to choosing a doctor. They often just ask a friend for a name and feel relieved if the doctor recommended still accepts new patients. Others never make the choice at all. Instead, they walk into the nearest clinic having no idea of the quality of the physician who will treat them. How can anyone make such an important decision so carelessly? Would they spend so little time choosing a new car? Probably not. First, they would read about different types of cars and would decide which model they wanted. Next, they would compare prices at different dealerships. Finally, they would test-drive several before making a purchase. Why do some people so often spend more time choosing their cars than their doctors? It is probably because they don't fully realize how doctors differ, nor do they know how to go about selecting the best one.

Just as in choosing a car, it takes time and effort to find a good doctor. That's why it's a good idea to choose your doctor when you are well. This allows you to be more objective and less frantic in your selection. Below we list

many of the different sources available and explain how
to use them effectively. If you follow these guidelines, we
feel confident that you will find an excellent doctor, someone you will want as your personal physician.

M e d i c a l   S o c i e t y

A good way to begin looking for a doctor is to call your
local medical society. Most larger cities have a medical
society (for example, the Atlanta Medical Society, San
Francisco Medical Society) to promote health care in the
community. The city's doctors make up its membership.
Although the society will not recommend one doctor over
another, it can provide a list of doctors who are taking
new patients and are located in your area. The society can
also answer your questions about the doctor's qualifications. Qualifications include such things as the medical
school and residency program the doctor attended, her
hospital affiliations, and her board certifications.

Although excellent medical schools are found throughout the world, it is easier to be certain of the quality of
the school if it is found in the United States or Canada
because it must adhere to strict guidelines to be accred-
ited. As with any type of professional schooling, some
programs may be considered better than others, but
nearly all provide an excellent medical education.

The residency program refers to the in-hospital training or internship a doctor receives after graduation from
medical school. During residency, the doctor is responsible for taking care of patients but is still supervised by
other doctors. The best residency programs are in hospitals affiliated with a medical university. A university hospital is more likely than a local hospital to have a wider
diversity of patients, because it is usually a referral center
for difficult cases. It will also have a stronger teaching

program than a community hospital because of the many university professors on staff.

Board certification means the primary-care doctor has passed a comprehensive written examination on general medical information. The examination is prepared by either the American Board of Internal Medicine or the American Board of Family Practice. A doctor typically takes this test after completing residency. Not all states require practicing physicians to be board certified. Board certification alone does not guarantee a fully capable doctor. It does serve as a good indication that your prospective doctor was trained well enough to pass a comprehensive written examination of her medical knowledge.

Questions to Ask the Medical Society

1. Can you give me a list of doctors in my area who are accepting new patients?
2. What medical school did she attend?
3. Where did she do her residency?
4. Is this hospital affiliated with a medical university?
5. Is she board certified?
6. Has she ever been disciplined by the State Medical Board or lost a malpractice suit?

Friend

Most people use a friend's advice to pick a doctor. This can be a very good source, because your information comes from someone you know and presumably trust. On the other hand, you must determine the basis of your friend's recommendation in order to decide how valuable it is. It must be based on more than just the doctor's personality. Understanding the things your friend considers to be important in a doctor, and matching those with the things *you* consider important will help you to determine how appropriate the recommended doctor would be for you.

Questions to Ask a Friend

1. Why do you recommend this doctor?
2. Do you feel that he is thorough?
3. Is there anything you don't like about him?
4. Do you trust his judgment?
5. Is he easy to talk to and does he seem concerned?
6. Does he explain your illnesses or problems and discuss how to treat them?
7. Do you feel rushed in his office?
8. Is it difficult to get an appointment?

Doctors

Another excellent source to help you choose a physician is another doctor. The source is best if the recommendation is based on more than just personal friendship. Another doctor is in a position to give you the type of advice you can get nowhere else. She can speak authoritatively about the clinical judgment and diagnostic skills of the physician she recommends.

It may be difficult to get a doctor's true opinion, because it is rare for one doctor to criticize another. If you ask one doctor what she thinks of another doctor you are considering, it is unlikely she would say anything negative. A better alternative for getting the information you want is to ask for a list of good doctors. If you already have the name of a doctor, you can see if it is on the list. If it isn't, you can then ask the doctor about the one in whom you are interested. Realize, however, that her assessment may be less than candid. You can tell a lot from the way she reacts to your question. Does she enthusiastically endorse your choice or just agree that he's "okay"?

Even when you don't know another doctor personally (for example, if you've just moved to a new city), there is a novel way to get a qualified doctor's advice. Call a locally respected hospital and ask for the name of the chief of internal medicine or family practice. Then call him, explain your circumstances, and ask if he is willing to help you find a doctor.

Questions to Ask Doctors

1. Who are the primary-care doctors whose *diagnostic skills* and *clinical judgment* most impress you?
2. Have you ever worked with this doctor personally?
3. Have you referred other patients to this doctor? What did they think of him?
4. The doctor I am considering trained at _____ medical school and did his residency at _____. Do you feel these are high-quality training programs?

Nurses

Hospital nurses are a valuable source of information if they have worked with the doctor in a clinical situation. Many hospitals now offer call-in nurse referrals (for example, Ask a Nurse) for doctors associated with that hospital. Nurses can comment on how committed a doctor is to patients and how well he interacts with them. Nurses are also more at liberty than a fellow doctor to tell you what they don't like. Ask a nurse the following questions.

Questions to Ask a Nurse

1. Have you worked with the doctor you've recommended?
2. Does this doctor seem committed to patients?
3. Is there anything about this doctor you don't like?
4. Would you personally want this doctor to care for you?

Doctor's Office

After you have narrowed your list, you can also get more information from a simple telephone call to the prospective doctor's office. By asking the right questions, you can learn a lot about the level of care provided there. Some of you may feel uncomfortable making a call like this. Don't. Your choice of doctor is too important to allow embarrassment or timidity to prevent you from getting this essential information. First, ask the receptionist if the doctor is accepting new patients. If she is, then ask the following questions.

Questions for the Doctor's Receptionist

1. Will I see my own doctor each time I come to the office? (This is a good question if you call a doctor who is in practice with a group of doctors. You will get better continuing care if you see the same doctor on each visit.)
2. How many patients does the doctor see in a typical day? (You are unlikely to receive adequate time from a doctor who sees more than twenty-five to thirty patients a day.)
3. How much advance notice must I give to schedule a routine physical exam? (If it takes more than a

couple months to schedule a complete physical, the doctor already has enough patients.)

4. How much time is set aside for a complete physical examination? (A thorough complete physical exam should take approximately one hour.)

5. How much time is scheduled for a routine office visit? (A routine office visit should be approximately fifteen minutes long.)

6. Is there twenty-four-hour coverage by the doctor or an associate? (Twenty-four-hour coverage is a must.)

7. If I require hospitalization will my own doctor care for me? (You want a doctor who is qualified to care for you if you require hospitalization.)

8. Does the doctor have ICU (intensive care unit) privileges in the hospital? (You want a doctor who is qualified to care for you if you become critically ill.)

9. At what hospital(s) does the doctor have admitting privileges? (You want to be certain the doctor you choose can admit you to the hospital you prefer.)

10. What are the charges for a complete exam and a routine office visit? (Cost is a frequent concern. Discuss insurance coverage or other individual needs with the doctor or receptionist before you are seen. Cost alone, however, is not indicative of the quality of a doctor's services.)

We also feel it is a good idea to visit a doctor's office before you commit yourself to becoming a patient. By far the best way to do this is to schedule an introductory office visit. This would not be a comprehensive exam, just a visit to get acquainted. Let the receptionist know that your purpose is to meet the doctor. We understand you may feel too anxious or awkward to do this. Here again, if you can overcome your reservations, the information you can obtain is well worth any temporary uneasiness. Remember, your health for years to come can be directly affected by the doctor you choose. We also understand that some doctors might deny the request for this type of visit. Perhaps those that do already have enough patients.

An introductory visit allows you to meet the doctor in a relaxed setting and get to know him before medical problems arise. Even though there is more to good medical care than interpersonal skills, you want to find a doctor whose personality doesn't conflict with your own. Before you visit, decide what type of doctor you want and what type of patient you are. Are you someone who wants all of the facts and to be intimately involved with decision making? Or are you someone who prefers to let the doctor make the choices for you? You can discuss this with the doctor during the visit. Let him know about any particular fears or concerns you have (fear of needles, vegetarian diet, etc.).

During this initial visit, you also can ask questions that are pertinent to your future health care. While you wait, you can see the waiting room and how many patients are waiting to be seen. You might ask some of them questions about the doctor and staff.

Below we outline some questions to ask the doctor during your visit. Understand that an introductory visit is a new experience for most doctors. Explain your purpose and show that you are sincere. The responses should be sincere as well. If they are not, it's better to know now rather than later.

Questions to Ask During the Introductory Visit

1. How do you feel about this introductory meeting?
2. Why do you practice primary-care medicine?
3. What are some of the things about being a doctor that you wish patients understood?
4. What is your opinion about periodic examinations?

5. If I were to require hospitalization, would you be the one taking care of me?
6. How would you describe your knowledge of my chronic problem (if applicable) or of my age group?
7. I am changing doctors because . . . (if applicable).

A Word About HMOs

A number of you may belong to or are considering joining a health maintenance organization (HMO). Although there are many types, an HMO is essentially an organization developed by insurance companies that enables you to receive medical services from a certain group of doctors for a predetermined fee. Although your ability to select a physician would be restricted to the list of doctors participating in the HMO, you can still apply the information from this chapter to choose your physician.

All of the sources we've described should help in your search for a good primary-care physician. The more people you talk to, the more complete a picture you will have of your future doctor. As you have seen, the selection of a good doctor can be done in a planned and orderly way. There are things you can do and questions you can ask to maximize the probability that your doctor will be one with respected clinical as well as interpersonal skills. This knowledge is the first step toward the development of the kind of relationship you want with your doctor—one based on trust and respect. Your relationship with your doctor can be the most intimate and long-lasting professional encounter you ever have. In the next chapter, we will look at ways to assess your present medical care if you already have a primary-care physician.

3

How to Know if You Have a Good Doctor

Webster's *Collegiate Dictionary* defines a doctor as "someone licensed to practice medicine." We define a *good* doctor as one who is committed to practice medicine to the best of his ability. Now that you know why it is important to have a good doctor, we will show you how to recognize one.

For some patients, a good doctor is one who seems to care about them. Caring is essential in a doctor; a doctor who lacks a caring attitude is undesirable regardless of how much medical knowledge he has. On the other hand, there is more to an excellent physician than a good bedside manner. You want a doctor who is meticulous when he questions you about your symptoms, performs examinations carefully, takes time to discuss conclusions, and is a knowledgeable and skilled diagnostician. Being a good doctor has as much to do with the attitude toward and commitment to the practice of medicine as with having a set of specific skills. Because of the importance of this concept, we avoid presenting the information in this chapter in the form of rules or checklists. There are definite points you can attend to, but keep the total picture in mind as you think about your own doctor.

Some of these points will be easier than others for you to evaluate. Fortunately, the doctor with most of these characteristics is likely to have all of them.

C a r i n g

It is extremely important that your doctor make you feel she cares about you. Admittedly, this is a subjective judgment based as much on your expectations as on the doctor's actual behavior. Some doctors will be more skilled in public relations than others. Some may care about you very much but not be very good at making small talk. Try to think of a caring doctor as one who respects you and shows that respect by listening carefully, trying to make you feel comfortable, and responding to your questions with patience. She is genuinely concerned that you have a clear understanding of what she is doing or recommending and why; she wants you to be an informed and participating patient. Sometimes small things the doctor does make you feel as if she cares—such as calling you herself about abnormal test results. A caring doctor will almost certainly show compassion and concern if something serious develops. She will think of you and your reactions as she presents you with information about a major illness and discusses its treatment. Of course, different doctors display their compassion in different ways, but a compassionate doctor is likely to provide strong emotional support because she truly cares.

T h o r o u g h n e s s

When you leave your doctor's office, you want to leave with the feeling that he has done a careful and thorough investigation of your complaints. A thorough doctor is one who doesn't want to miss a diagnosis because he has failed to make the appropriate effort. As you will see below, this characteristic applies to all clinical aspects of the doctor's responsibilities.

The Office Interview

The doctor interviews you to determine the exact nature of your symptoms. He should do whatever is necessary to get a clear and accurate picture of what you are trying to describe. A thorough doctor will give you the opportunity to say everything you want to say related to a symptom you have been experiencing. This doesn't necessarily mean he won't interrupt you. It does mean his interruptions are for clarification or redirection, not to rush you along. He also will ask you his own questions about your symptoms. To be thorough, he must ask questions to make sure he understands exactly what you've noticed.

The Physical Examination

A good doctor will give a thorough examination of the areas suggested by your description of symptoms. Even though you can't know if she examines the appropriate areas, you can follow the logical progression of the exam. The doctor should give you the feeling she is taking her time performing the exam. A good time to pay attention is during a complete physical examination. The actual exam of your body should take at least twenty minutes and should be performed by the doctor rather than by an assistant. During a complete examination, the doctor should do the procedures that take a little more time, such as listening to your heart in both the sitting and lying positions, and performing a rectal exam. A woman should have an unhurried breast examination and a Pap smear. The doctor should also discuss with her current recommendations for mammograms. A thorough doctor will always discuss her findings and recommendations at the conclusion of the physical examination.

Explanation and Patient Education

A common thread throughout this book is the importance of your learning more about your medical care. A thorough doctor takes extra effort to explain his reasoning because he wants his patients to understand. He knows an informed patient is more likely to feel comfortable with his judgment and is less likely to worry needlessly. He explains the risks involved in testing, the side effects of treatments, and expected results. A thorough doctor will not knowingly let a patient walk out of his office who does not understand why he recommends a certain test or what the results of the test could mean.

Current Knowledge

Everyone wants a doctor who knows everything and learns every piece of new medical information as soon as it comes out. Nobody has one. It is possible, however, to have a doctor who was well trained and who continues to learn and apply medical advances that have taken place since his graduation. This important quality, unfortunately, is the most difficult one for you to judge. If your doctor was trained at a university medical center and is board certified, you can surmise that he was well trained. If you chose your doctor by asking for recommendations from nurses or other doctors, you will know that your doctor is respected in the medical community.

The best way for you to try to assess your doctor's knowledge is when he discusses his conclusions with you.

Having a knowledgeable doctor does not mean you will receive a ready diagnosis for every minor complaint. It does mean that when he discusses the reasons for his decisions and recommendations, they sound logical and well thought out.

There may be occasions when you discuss with your doctor particular treatments you have read about in magazines or seen on television. Your doctor may seem to dismiss such treatments. Don't be surprised if your doctor has this reaction. This is not necessarily an indication of your doctor's lack of medical knowledge or willingness to learn. The popular media frequently cover treatments that have not been supported by research and, consequently, do not have the support of your physician. On the other hand, a knowledgeable doctor doesn't make you feel foolish for asking and will give you good reasons for his opinions.

Complete Records

Thorough continuing care requires the maintenance of good records. A doctor has too many patients to rely on memory alone. Records are the doctor's only means for recognizing and using previous knowledge about you and any illnesses you might have had. You probably will not have access to your doctor's records of your visits. Even if you did, it would be difficult for you to determine how good they were, because you wouldn't have a basis for comparison. Your doctor's notes should include a record of office visits—when they were, what your symptoms were, what the diagnosis was (if one was reached), and any prescribed treatment. See figure 1 for a sample chart entry.

Because one of the reasons you have a primary-care physician is the diagnostic advantage of seeing the same doctor over time, he should have access to information

---

Figure 1

Sample Chart Entry

S) Complains of burning with urination for the last week. Also urinating more frequently. Has had mild back pain for two days. Felt "feverish" last night. Never has had a kidney stone.

O) Temperature—100. Abdominal exam negative. Back with mild tenderness in area of right kidney. Urine specimen shows many pus cells and bacteria.

A) Suspect urinary infection. Feel that back pain suggests kidney involvement rather than simple bladder infection. Feel that pain is not severe enough to suggest a kidney stone.

P) Culture urine specimen. Will treat with antibiotic for full two weeks because of likely kidney involvement. Patient is to call if fever is higher than 101. Recheck specimen in one week.

S) The *subjective* symptoms described by the patient.
O) The *objective* findings detected by the doctor.
A) The doctor's *assessment* of what he thinks is the patient's problem.
P) The doctor's *plan* for how he will treat the patient's problem.

---

from previous visits. When you visit your doctor for a follow-up appointment, therefore, he should know why you are there. Thorough records should also document all important information related to your past medical care. Consequently, your doctor should request medical records from other physicians you've had in the past. Records should include all tests the doctor has ordered for you, when and why they were ordered, and the results. Your doctor should be able to give you a definite reason for ordering the same test you've had in the recent past. Finally, good records should include a complete listing of the medications you take and any allergic reactions you've experienced. When you compare your list with your doctor's, they should agree.

Health Maintenance

A thorough primary-care doctor wants to help you maintain good health. She takes extra time to inquire about your health habits, particularly if she sees evidence of change over time, such as consistent weight gain or rises in your cholesterol level. If you have a specific habit (smoking) or characteristic of your life-style (stress) that should be modified, she will discuss why changes are recommended and how they can be achieved. At first, this may not be your favorite facet of a good doctor, but you should appreciate her concern. If you have a chronic problem, such as hypertension or diabetes, she will see you periodically to follow its course to prevent future health problems. She will also review your medications with you to make sure you take them correctly.

Availability

Serious medical problems can occur at unpredictable times, which means you want a doctor who is available when you need him. You should always have access to your doctor or his associate during an emergency. When you call your doctor because of a true emergency, he should call you back promptly. If you call during office hours with a less serious problem, you should assume your doctor is busy with other patients. He may not be able to call you immediately, but later in the day he should return your calls. Your doctor should also have an answering service to take after-hours calls.

Possible Causes for Misunderstanding in a Good Doctor-Patient Relationship

Because the relationship with your doctor is one that develops over time, the most accurate picture of him is one that rests on his usual performance. It is likely there will be an occasion or two when you are not completely satisfied with a visit to your doctor. You may feel he was less concerned or attentive than usual, and you may be irritated or hurt because of it. We have just stressed the importance of a caring and knowledgeable doctor. Although a possible source of concern, isolated incidents should not usually be used to determine the quality of your doctor. Sometimes situations that seem irritating result from reasons other than an uncaring doctor. We all have bad days at work. Our purpose is to provide you with a little more insight into your doctor's role and to encourage you to assess his *typical* behavior. We hope you will use this information to open the lines of communication with your doctor and discuss with him minor or occasional annoyances that have the potential of disrupting an otherwise good relationship.

One concern you might have is an extremely long wait in the doctor's waiting room. When a good doctor establishes his daily schedule, he has every intention of moving through his day by sticking as closely as possible to his schedule. Typically, there should not be lengthy waits associated with your visits. Occasionally, however, both your schedule and the doctor's schedule can be disrupted by an emergency call or the arrival of a suddenly ill patient. This could result in a longer patient evaluation than anticipated or even the need for the physician to go to the hospital to admit the patient. There also is the possibility that your doctor has spent more time than planned with a patient explaining an abnormal test result or discussing a serious diagnosis. A thorough doctor will take the time necessary to review the situation with the patient and provide emotional support. Clearly, occurrences such as these may possibly result in long delays for the remainder of the day. If your delay is exceedingly long, you should expect to be told why.

There also may be an occasion when you are less than satisfied with your doctor's attitude. If you have a good relationship and expect a certain level of attention, you might be very aware if your doctor seems a bit preoccupied or more abrupt than usual. You may be offended or hurt if this happens and think the doctor doesn't care as much as you thought he did. If you have a visit like this, keep in mind that this reaction may not actually reflect a lack of concern. A doctor sees many patients each day. It is sometimes difficult for him to "switch gears" continuously as he listens to each patient's symptoms. He must try to reorient his thinking as he deals with each case separately. He must always attempt to consider only the case before him and not allow his concentration to be distracted by an earlier case. On occasion, however, it is difficult for him to move on to the next patient if he is still worried about the person he has just seen. A good doctor should always give you the medical care you need, but there could be an instance when it is difficult for him to erase immediately his concern for another patient. The result may be that even a good doctor could seem less social than usual.

A visit characterized by an unusually abrupt or intense interaction can also be disturbing. You may feel the doctor is being short with you, interrupting you, or asking a deluge of questions. A good doctor will not act this way on a regular basis. If it happens on a particular visit, consider the possibility of a frustrated physician trying to get a clear idea of the problems you have noticed. A casual or inarticulate presentation of symptoms may leave the doctor with only a vague impression of what you have been experiencing. She may, on occasion, overreact to that frustration, particularly if she is concerned about a serious cause for what you have told her. Even if you don't provide the doctor with the detailed information she needs, ultimately she is responsible for the accurate diagnosis of the problem. Neither you nor the doctor can accept or tolerate mistakes. As a result, and as you would expect, the doctor will be determined to get as much clarifying information as she can.

In this chapter, we have looked at the skills, behaviors, and attitudes of caring and thorough physicians. The many points we've presented should help you see how difficult it is to be a good doctor. That is not an excuse for someone who performs poorly, but we hope you will appreciate someone who does it well. As an informed patient, you are now in a better position to recognize your own doctor's abilities.

We don't insist that a doctor must follow all these guidelines to perform his job effectively. If you're quite happy with your present doctor, don't necessarily use this information to convince yourself otherwise. It is likely that your present opinion is correct and you should allow misgivings only if you discover significant factors that in the past you had never thought to question. Think about the qualities your doctor has that you consider special. Would you recommend him to friends without reservation? If so, for what reasons? The answers to these questions form the basis of your present opinion. On the other hand, if you are already a bit uneasy or dissatisfied with your present doctor, you can use this information to decide if your suspicions are well founded.

Unfortunately, you may have had a series of experiences with your doctor that have lessened your trust in his abilities or have prevented or damaged a positive relationship with him. There are instances when changing doctors is the best course of action. In the next chapter, we will look at some of the things that might indicate the need for you to look for another primary-care physician.

4

Why to Change Doctors

S ome patients would never consider changing doctors. Even when they have begun to feel uneasy about their doctors' medical judgments, they find it too hard to leave people they have confided in for so long. Instead, they continue to see doctors they no longer fully trust. Still other patients take changing doctors too lightly. They jump from one doctor to another, always in search of the one who will fulfill all their expectations. They continuously scrutinize each new doctor, always on the lookout for any evidence that proves this doctor is no better than the last.

There are times when it is best to find a new doctor. There are other times when the problem is actually one of unrealistic expectations. So, when is it appropriate to change? Certainly, when your doctor is unable to meet your reasonable expectations. We cannot assume to know what is most important to you, but we can outline the basic expectations all patients should have of their physicians. Our purpose is to emphasize specific points that should be a definite cause for concern. If you use each point presented earlier to judge your doctor, you may well become overly critical. If, however, your doctor fails to meet the fundamental professional expectations in some of the ways we describe below, you should consider the possibility that this doctor may not be best for you. We have stressed the importance of looking at the *overall performance* of your doctor before making such a major decision. The expectations you have of your physician can be grouped under the areas of communication and medical judgment.

Failure to Communicate

The ability to talk comfortably with your doctor is the cornerstone of a good relationship. So much of what a doctor does depends on dialogue. If you find that you and your doctor can no longer discuss matters easily, this is a serious problem that, if left uncorrected, can compromise your care. Below we pose some questions that represent examples of failed communication.

1. Is your doctor unsympathetic, intimidating, or condescending? It is essential that you feel your doctor truly cares about you. Otherwise, you will never fully trust his motives. If your doctor repeatedly makes you feel foolish or uneasy, you should seriously consider changing doctors.
2. Does your doctor fail to answer your questions? Your doctor should make an effort to answer your questions. The time allocated for an office visit should provide ample opportunity for the doctor to address a reasonable number of questions. If he repeatedly ignores or glosses over them, then you should be justifiably disturbed.

3. Does your doctor always give you a prescription without ever discussing your problem? Your doctor should try to tell you what he thinks your problem is and how the medication he prescribes will help. His typical procedure for discussing the effects of treatment should allow you to understand what to expect and how to take the medication safely and effectively. It is not adequate for the doctor to write a prescription, tell you to take it, and walk out of the room.

4. Does your doctor criticize your wishes for another opinion? You should feel free to get another doctor's opinion if you want one. It is normal for your doctor to ask what you expect from another doctor's input, but he should not respond to your request with anger or condescending remarks.

5. Is your doctor inaccessible? Must you always get your answers from his nurse? Obviously, you should be able to contact your doctor or his associate during an emergency. You should also be allowed to discuss less serious problems with him if you feel his nurse can't answer your questions adequately. Ask yourself if your calls actually required speaking directly with the doctor. A nurse can handle many of the numerous phone calls a doctor receives each day. For example, it is appropriate for a nurse to answer a question about how long to take a medicine if she first discussed it with the doctor. If your doctor never returns phone calls for legitimate requests, such as if you are experiencing an allergic reaction to a medication, you have a right to feel slighted.

Inadequate Medical Judgment

Medical judgment is more than just a knowledge of medical facts. It is the ability to use medical knowledge to make appropriate decisions. Unless you feel confident about your doctor's medical judgment, you will always feel a bit uneasy with her recommendations. Assessing your doctor's medical judgment is difficult. If you pay attention to how she evaluates your problems, however, you can get a good idea about it. Below we point out some of the clues to a less careful physician.

1. Your doctor rarely examines you when you complain of a symptom.

   You should expect the doctor to examine you after a complaint of a specific problem or discomfort, because the physical exam is one of the ways a doctor confirms or rules out possible diagnoses suggested by your symptoms. If she repeatedly gives you an opinion without an examination, you have a legitimate reason to question it.

2. Your doctor repeatedly gives you a prescription without asking further questions or examining you.

   A doctor should give treatment for a problem only after considering its possible causes. Otherwise, improper treatment of symptoms could allow the disease to progress. Even when a definitive diagnosis is not made (as in the case of a muscle ache in the arm), the doctor must explore carefully possible reasons for the pain before she feels comfortable prescribing medication to relieve it.

3. She repeatedly orders the same X ray, even though you have had the same one recently.

   Doctors use tests to help confirm diagnostic possibilities and sometimes repeat testing is needed to follow an illness to its resolution. (For example, if you had an X ray that showed pneumonia, you would need another one shortly after treatment to be certain the illness had been cured.)

   Some less careful physicians, however, may quickly

order tests as a substitute for a more complete initial exam. If you find yourself getting another X ray with every complaint, you should wonder about your doctor's thoroughness and the quality of his records.

4. She repeatedly sends you to specialists for even minor complaints.

Doctors often use specialists to confirm their suspicions of serious illness, help them with a difficult diagnostic problem, or perform a sophisticated diagnostic test. Some doctors use specialists much more frequently because they are unsure about their own clinical judgment. If your doctor sends you to see someone else for almost every minor complaint, you may have reason to question her judgment. Understand, a symptom that seems minor to you could have more significance to your doctor. Don't let your doctor's *occasional* need for a second opinion cause you immediately to question her competence.

5. An assistant rather than the doctor is the one you usually see.

A doctor with good medical judgment knows that many of the abnormal signs found during a physical examination are not obvious. She will feel confident that they are absent only if she conducts the examination herself. Your doctor, therefore, is the one who should perform your exams. It is appropriate for an assistant to perform several of the more straightforward procedures such as taking your blood pressure, checking your vision, or recording your temperature.

Remember, just as in choosing a doctor, deciding to change to another one should be a major decision. It should be based on her usual or typical interaction with you. You shouldn't let an isolated minor misunderstanding alter an otherwise good relationship. Like anyone

else, your doctor might just have been having a bad day.
Talk about your concerns. You may find she's more receptive to your feelings than you thought. If you find that an
open discussion still doesn't clear the air, you will feel
more comfortable and justified with your decision to
change.

5

The Diagnosis

When you don't feel well and call the doctor you expect certain things. First, you expect the doctor to determine the cause of your illness or pain. Second, you expect to receive treatment to relieve any discomfort you are feeling. The first expectation is called receiving a diagnosis—the doctor identifies the source of the problem or the reason for the pain.

It's important for you to realize that a diagnosis, per se, is not the inevitable result of an examination. If your doctor cannot give you a diagnosis, it doesn't necessarily mean that there is something mysterious wrong with you or that your doctor is incompetent. In fact, recent research has shown more than 70 percent of all common symptoms presented by patients to their doctors are never diagnosed because they simply do not represent disease (Kroenke et al., 1989). Instead, they are nonspecific aches or pains that are either normal bodily sensations or muscle pulls or strains. Your body can have a fleeting discomfort that doesn't necessarily mean something is wrong. Of course, there are many symptoms that do represent a problem. When that's the case, you want the doctor to be able to diagnose the cause.

Arriving at a diagnosis can sometimes be difficult, even though the process itself is actually quite straightforward. The doctor follows a specific sequence of steps as she gathers information from a variety of sources. First, she interviews you and asks you to describe any discomforts (your symptoms). Then the doctor examines the appropriate areas of your body. Finally, she orders any necessary tests. As she receives information from each of these sources, the doctor stops to analyze the data and determine if continued assessment is needed. At any stage, she may conclude that she has sufficient information to determine the cause of the problem.

The ease with which a doctor makes a diagnosis will depend on the nature of the illness and the symptoms it produces. Sometimes these symptoms are so typical that the diagnosis is both rapid and certain. All that is required are a few questions and a simple exam. Unfortunately, not all diagnoses are so easy. Some symptoms are much less specific and could require more extensive investigation. A good example of this type of symptom is chronic fatigue. Although the usual cause of fatigue is poor physical conditioning or insufficient sleep, it is also possible it could result from a more serious underlying cause such as depression, cancer, infection, anemia, or hormonal deficiency.

The remainder of this chapter presents a general overview of the diagnostic process. Once you understand this process, you will understand the importance of your participation in it. The extent to which you can participate will vary with each step. For example, the first step, the interview, consists primarily of your input. What you say or do not say has a great effect on your doctor's subsequent evaluation and can have tremendous consequences for you. On the other hand, the physical exam will not require much participation on your part. Remember, our purpose is not to teach you how to diagnose yourself.

Rather, we are trying to give you an understanding of the reasoning process used by your doctor. By becoming familiar with this you will soon see how much you can do to help.

Overview of Diagnostic Process

The first step of the diagnostic process is the patient interview. Despite all of the sophisticated diagnostic tests now available, the information you give your doctor remains the most important aspect of the diagnostic process. The symptoms you describe determine the possible disorders your doctor considers and influence nearly all his subsequent actions. Initially, as you begin to describe your discomfort, the doctor listens just to get the big picture. He prompts you to remember all the symptoms you have experienced. As he thinks about the information you are giving him, he constantly makes decisions about the relevance and irrelevance of what you are describing.

The doctor next attempts to match your symptoms with those associated with diseases familiar to him. As he asks more specific questions, some diseases will appear more or less likely, and some he can eliminate altogether (see figure 2). This may be a difficult process when the classic or textbook symptoms of certain diseases are different from those actually experienced by a patient with that illness. The words a patient uses to describe a symptom also are very important. For example, a patient says that he has been experiencing "dizziness." This word may be used to describe (1) a whirling sensation as if the room is spinning around, (2) a feeling of imbalance or unsteadiness in walking, or (3) a lightheaded or faint feeling. Each of these feelings is quite distinct and may result from *very different causes*. Even a very subtle difference in

---

Figure 2

Possible Causes of Leg Pain

Patient's Complaint: "My leg hurts."

Diagnoses Considered:

1. Muscle strain
2. Clot in vein (phlebitis)
3. Pressure on nerve from disc in back (sciatica)
4. Narrowed artery (poor circulation)
5. Pressure on nerve from arthritis (spinal stenosis)

	Diagnosis Excluded	**Reason**
Q. How long? A. 2 months	1. Muscle strain	Unlikely would last that long
Q. Where in your leg? A. In the back of my thigh	2. Clot in vein	Pain usually in calf
Q. How long does it last? A. 10–15 minutes	3. Disc in back	Pain usually lasts longer
Q. Does walking worsen it? A. No	4. Narrowed artery	Pain of poor circulation typically gets worse with exercise
Doctor suspects probable cause is pressure on nerve from arthritis (spinal stenosis)		Further questions reveal that the pain occurs when patient stands and improves when he sits down, qualities typical of spinal stenosis

the symptom you describe can suggest a very different cause (see figure 3). The way you describe what you feel can have a significant effect on how long it takes your doctor to find the source of the problem and could even cause him to miss the diagnosis altogether. Once the doctor has a clear picture of your symptoms and has narrowed the range of possible diagnoses, he knows where to concentrate his physical examination.

The physical examination is the doctor's hands-on inspection of the body. During the physical exam, the doctor looks for more clues to narrow further the list of pos-

---

Figure 3

Numbness in the Fingers

**Fingers Involved
(shaded areas)**   **Likely Cause**

Pressure on nerve in wrist

Pressure on nerve in elbow

Pressure on nerve in neck

Possible causes of numbness in fingers; entirely different causes are suggested by very subtle differences.

sible diagnoses. If the interview was fruitful, the doctor already has some idea of what he is looking for during the exam. For example, if you complain of pain in the upper right side of your abdomen, the doctor will consider abnormalities of the gallbladder, liver, kidney, and intestines. He has already attempted to determine which organ is responsible for your symptom by further questioning. His subsequent findings during the physical examination will help with this decision (see figure 4). Although the doctor will be following a type of blueprint during the physical examination, it is important for him always to remain alert for the unexpected because it could cause him to reformulate his diagnosis. Not only must the doctor detect any abnormalities during the physical exam, he must realize the significance of the ab-

---

Figure 4

Physical Findings with Abdominal Pain

	Usual Type of Pain	Possible Findings on Physical Exam
Gallbladder	Deep, severe ache lasting several hours	Tenderness below rib cage on right
Liver	Often painless. Sometimes dull and steady, worse with deep breath	Enlargement below rib cage on right
Kidney	Usually intense and continuous	Tender in the back
Intestine	Cramping and intermittent	Generalized tenderness throughout the abdomen

normalities he finds. Sometimes the relationship between the symptoms, the physical findings, and the cause is obvious. The problem is solved and no further clarification is required. In other instances, more information is needed. If so, the doctor begins the third information-gathering stage of the diagnostic process—the ordering of appropriate laboratory studies and diagnostic tests.

Diagnostic tests can be simple or complex. Simple laboratory tests include routine blood and urine studies, chest X rays, and electrocardiograms. Frequently, the doctor will use these tests as supporting evidence for the diagnosis he considers most likely. He also can use simple laboratory tests to rule out a less likely diagnosis. For example, a normal chest X ray can rule out pneumonia.

Complex tests include more elaborate procedures such as specialized X rays, scans, or biopsies. Many of these tests are expensive, some can be painful, and a few pose some risk to the patient. Because of these concerns, the doctor must have a clear and valid reason for ordering them, such as the severity of the symptom or the seriousness of the diagnosis considered. Some symptoms demand an explanation even if they occur only once. For example, if you ever see blood in your urine, the doctor must test until he discovers the source of the problem. Possible causes include infection, a stone, or a tumor. Other symptoms, however, require explanations only when they persist. Your doctor may wait to determine if a symptom such as diarrhea will continue over time before ordering further tests. In fact, the extent of testing often is determined by the patient's age, sex, and family history. For example, the possibility that one episode of blood on the stool represents a colon cancer is considerably less likely in a twenty-year-old than in a sixty-five-year-old patient. This fact alone affects the extent to which the symptom will be analyzed. If a simple rectal exam reveals hemorrhoids in both, the doctor may accept this as the probable cause of bleeding only in the younger patient. The older patient's age demands that the doctor also rule out a coexisting colon cancer by looking at the entire colon with appropriate tests.

Consequences of the Diagnostic Process

After your doctor has gone through all stages of the diagnostic process, one of two things will happen. Either the doctor will have a diagnosis or he won't. As we mentioned before, the absence of a diagnosis is not necessarily bad. Let's look at some possible consequences of the diagnostic process and discuss what they mean.

The doctor arrives at a diagnosis. In this instance, the physician has discovered that the symptoms you've described do fit the pattern of a disease, illness, or condition known to him. The physical examination and any tests administered have revealed findings that also fit this pattern. Your doctor may have made the diagnosis in five minutes or he may have needed several visits and several tests to determine the cause of your symptoms. Next, the doctor will recommend a course of treatment or discuss treatment options with you.

The doctor does not arrive at a diagnosis. There are two major reasons a doctor doesn't arrive at a diagnosis. The first is that the doctor did not find a definite cause for the problem or symptom because the symptoms did not represent disease or anything abnormal. As we've said, the complaint or symptom may be nothing more than a noticeable, normal body sensation. It also is possible the doctor was able to rule out a significant cause for the problem and can dismiss a serious diagnosis he considered originally. We present an example in figure 5.

The second reason the doctor may not arrive at a diag-

Figure 5

Absence of a Diagnosis

A middle-aged patient complains of several episodes of sharp chest pain each lasting a few seconds. The doctor needs no tests to decide whether this could be something serious. A few seconds of chest pain does *not* represent disease.

If, on the other hand, the patient had complained of chest tightness that lasted a few minutes, the doctor would have to consider heart-artery disease as a possible cause. He would ask further clarifying questions to help him decide. Does exercise bring it on? What relieves it? Is it associated with shortness of breath? He also would consider risk factors for heart disease such as whether the patient smoked, had elevated blood cholesterol, or had relatives with early heart disease.

These factors would all help determine the extent of the evaluation to rule out heart-artery blockage. The end result of the diagnostic work-up will be that the doctor either finds heart-artery disease is present or feels confident it is not. That is what is really important. It is not necessary for him to explain a few minutes of chest tightness if it does not represent heart disease. There really aren't any other serious causes.

nosis is that he was unable to find the cause of the problem even though one exists. He may simply have missed the diagnosis. A missed diagnosis may be the result of a lack of information (the physician didn't make the appropriate effort, is unfamiliar with the disease, has failed to detect an abnormal finding on the physical exam, or has not administered the appropriate test). A missed diagnosis can also be the result of misleading or incorrect infor-

Figure 6

Example of a Missed Diagnosis

The thyroid is a gland at the base of the neck, which secretes a hormone that regulates the body's metabolism. If the gland becomes overactive and secretes too much of this hormone, it speeds up the body's metabolism, causing the patient to become excessively nervous, to sweat excessively, and to lose weight. An overactive thyroid gland usually produces two abnormalities found upon physical examination—a rapid pulse and an enlarged thyroid gland.

Below we describe the evaluation of a patient who complains of "feeling nervous." The doctor could mistakenly diagnose the patient's problem as anxiety rather than an overactive thyroid gland at any step of the diagnostic process. Possible reasons include an insufficient interview, an inadequate physical exam, or an inappropriate conclusion.

1. *The doctor conducts an inadequate interview:* The doctor does not ask follow-up questions when the patient reports feeling nervous.
2. *The doctor does not consider the significance of an additional symptom reported by the patient:* The patient also reported the loss of twenty pounds.
3. *The doctor misses the diagnosis through a lack of effort, such as not conducting a physical exam:* The doctor did not examine the patient after learning she had lost twenty pounds and had been breaking into sweats.
4. *The doctor misses the diagnosis because he fails to detect an abnormal physical finding:* The doctor failed to detect the enlarged thyroid and rapid pulse rate.
5. *The doctor fails to consider the significance of an abnormal physical finding:* The doctor notices the rapid pulse but dismisses its importance and does not examine the thyroid.
6. *The doctor has all the necessary information but fails to piece it together correctly.* The doctor finds an enlarged thyroid and rapid pulse rate but still diagnoses anxiety.

mation (unusual symptoms, poorly identified symptoms, confusing lab results). Even when he has all the necessary information, he can still miss the diagnosis if he doesn't piece it together correctly. Your doctor cannot diagnose the disease you have unless he first considers it (see figure 6).

Your physician knows that, ultimately, he is responsible for a missed diagnosis regardless of the amount or quality of your input. You certainly can improve the chances for a rapid and accurate diagnosis, however, by carefully describing your symptoms. In the next chapter, we discuss how to prepare yourself for the interview portion of your visit to the doctor's office and provide guidelines for clear and straightforward communication.

6

The Interview

The patient interview is the most critical component of the diagnostic process and is the step most dependent on your participation. As we have noted earlier, the symptoms you describe will determine nearly everything else your doctor will do. Trying to put a personal experience such as pain into words can be difficult. You must realize, however, that the words you use to describe a feeling or type of pain will be the words the doctor uses to identify potential diagnoses. Because the same words may mean different things to different people, it is critical that both you and your doctor agree on the meaning of your words and how they represent what you feel. Patients have never been taught how to present this information clearly or to realize how important it is. A significant portion of this chapter is devoted to helping you learn how to present your symptoms in the clearest possible way. We will talk specifically about how to prepare for an office visit and how to interact with the doctor once you are there.

Preparation for the interview with your physician should begin as soon as the first major symptom appears. When you start to hurt or feel ill, a series of thoughts may enter your mind. You immediately begin to evaluate the pain, try to determine the cause, and decide whether the problem is serious enough to warrant seeing the doctor. There is no general guideline or rule of thumb to help you make this decision. If the symptom continues to occur, is particularly painful, or is simply causing you enough concern to make you consider seeing a doctor, then calling your physician is probably the best idea. Once you decide to make an appointment, do *not* continue to dwell on whether your visit is necessary. Now is the time to turn your attention to the symptom or symptoms you've noticed and observe the specific characteristics of the problem.

It may be hard for you to know where to focus your attention. How are you to know what is important? Below we present specific guidelines to help solve this problem. Not only does this outline tell you what to look for, it helps you describe your symptoms to your doctor. Why do you need an outline like this one? Everyone, at one time or another, has forgotten to tell the doctor about a symptom, or spent a good portion of an office visit trying to remember an important point such as when the pain started or how long it lasted. It's easy to feel disoriented, timid, or embarrassed while you are in the doctor's office, and, consequently, you may become confused about what you are trying to say. The typical office visit is approximately fifteen minutes long. Given that fact, it is good to know that by preparing a thorough description of your symptoms you can make the most effective use of your time with the doctor.

This outline will guide you through the initial presentation of symptoms to your doctor. The questions are posed to represent the most logical order of presentation. It's best to answer the questions at home and bring in your responses. Figure 7 provides you with an illustration of how this outline can work.

Figure 7

Describing Symptoms (Headache)

When

When did you first notice the problem? "Several months ago."

Where

Where on your body is the problem located? "At the back of my neck and my temples."

How

How does it feel? "It's a dull ache."
How often does the problem occur? "Nearly every day."
How long does it last each time it occurs? "It lasts for several hours."

What

What brings the problem on or makes it worse? "Maybe studying."
What relieves the problem? "I've tried aspirin, but it didn't help much."
What else do you notice with it? "Nothing."

Why

Why are you concerned? "I want to be sure it's not something serious like a tumor."

Sample Presentation of Information

"Doctor, I've been having headaches for the last several months. They seem to start in the back of my neck, but later it also hurts in my temples. It's a dull ache that lasts several hours, usually until I go to bed. The headaches don't prevent me from studying but they do make it more difficult. I usually take a couple of aspirin, which eases the pain a little but doesn't make it go away. I have been under a lot of pressure recently because of exams, but I don't think that's causing them. What concerns me is that I don't usually have headaches. To be honest, I'm a little worried it might be something serious, like a brain tumor. My roommate's cousin died of one." (The doctor would probably ask other questions about blurred vision, nausea, medications, and whether the headaches were causing the patient to awaken from sleep.)

Describing Your Symptoms

When

1. *When did you first notice the problem?* (yesterday, a week ago, last year) The answer to this question should indicate when the problem *first began*, not when it became worse. Try to be precise.

Where

2. *Where on your body is the problem located?* (in my right shoulder, in my lower back) Be specific. A phrase such as "pain in the temples" is more descriptive than "headache." If possible, point to the body part or area.

How

3. *How does it feel?* (sharp—like a knife sticking; pressing—like a vise tightening; cramping—like a towel wringing) When giving a description, try to avoid including potentially misleading diagnostic elements, for example, "what an ulcer must feel like."
4. *How often does the problem occur?* (daily, a couple of times a week, continuously) If there is no distinct pattern, either give an average frequency or estimate how many times it has occurred since it began.
5. *How long does it last each time it occurs?* (a second, several minutes, several hours) Avoid phrases such as "a short while," which could mean a few seconds or a few minutes. Try to state specific amounts of time. If you don't know the time exactly, *estimate* it. This point is too critical to answer with "I don't know." Be careful to distinguish between descriptions such as "It lasts all day" and "It happens several times during the day." If the length of time varies for each occurrence, give a range: "The pain can last thirty minutes to several hours."

What

6. *What brings the problem on or makes it worse?* (exercise, hunger, anxiety) You could have several responses to this question. If the problem occurs at random, let the doctor know that nothing in particular precipitates it.
7. *What relieves the problem?* (aspirin, antacids, a heating pad) Describe anything that you have tried that has lessened or alleviated the pain or problem. You also would want to indicate what you've tried that hasn't helped.
8. *What else do you notice with it?* (dizziness, nausea, back pain) Describe any symptoms that seem to occur with the major problem or any that you've noticed have been occurring for about the same length of time.

Why

9. *Why do you think you are ill?* (I think I might have an ulcer. Do you think it could be something serious like a tumor?) The *conclusion* of the interview is the time for you to share with the doctor your thoughts about possible reasons for your pain, illness, or discomfort. You also may want to express any concerns you have about specific illnesses.

Figures 8–10 are examples of this outline in use. As you can see, not all of the items on the outline can be applied to every problem. Always answer those that are appropriate. Don't answer these questions as if you are taking a test. We just ask that you don't give up too easily. Give the best estimate you can. The answers to these questions are too important to neglect. With a little effort, you will be surprised how much you can recall about a symptom you've had in the past.

The manner in which you present your symptoms to the doctor also can have an impact on the diagnostic

Figure 8

Describing Symptoms (Cough)

When

When did you first notice the problem? "Two months ago."

Where

Where on your body is the problem located? NA

How

How does it feel? "Coughing spells."
How often does the problem occur? "On and off all day long—will cough for a few minutes, then I can go an hour or two when I'm okay. Then I start coughing again. I may have fifteen or twenty coughing spells a day."
How long does it last each time it occurs? "Several minutes at a time."

What

What brings on the problem or makes it worse? "I'm not sure—maybe the pollen."
What relieves the problem? "Cough syrup doesn't help."
What else do you notice with it? "I also seem more short of breath."

Why

Why are you concerned? "I smoke and want to be sure it's not lung cancer."

Figure 9

Describing Symptoms (Weight Loss)

When

When did you first notice the problem? "About six months ago."

Where

Where on your body is the problem located? "My whole body—I've lost thirty pounds."

How

How does it feel? NA
How often does the problem occur? NA
How long does it last each time it occurs? NA

What

What brings on the problem or makes it worse? NA
What relieves the problem? NA
What else do you notice with it? "My appetite is poor; I just don't like the taste of food. I'm more tired than I used to be. I just don't want to get out of bed in the morning. I don't hurt anywhere."

Why

Why are you concerned? "I want to be sure I don't have anything serious."

Figure 10

Describing Symptoms
(Dizziness)

When

When did you first notice the problem? "This morning."

Where

Where on your body is the problem located? NA

How

How does it feel? "Dizzy—like the room is spinning and I can't hold on."
How often does the problem occur? "Whenever I turn my head quickly—it's happened five or six times."
How long does it last each time it occurs? "Just a few seconds."

What

What brings on the problem or makes it worse? "Moving fast, turning my head."
What relieves the problem? NA
What else do you notice with it? "I get nauseated."

Why

Why are you concerned? "I want something to make it stop."

process. The most effective and straightforward way to present information is to use our outline to give a simple narrative (figure 7). Describe each symptom fully before going to another one. Use clear and direct words to describe how you feel. The doctor is likely to have follow-up questions and points to discuss. Because you have already reviewed your symptoms in detail, you will be able to answer his questions precisely and honestly.

There are several other important points to consider. There may be occasions when you are reluctant to mention a certain symptom or concern. Perhaps you assume the doctor would notice the problem if it were really important or would ask about it if it were a symptom of a significant illness. He might not, however, even consider the correct diagnosis if you don't mention all the corresponding symptoms. Other times you may fail to mention a symptom because you fear the possibility of future testing. For example, you may not mention chest pain because you fear it could be heart disease and might require expensive or painful tests. Realize that any future action will require your consent and participation, so just concentrate on taking one step at a time. Remember, when disease is there, you want your doctor to find it. Apprehension or fear also might cause you to present in an offhand way or otherwise minimize certain symptoms ("I have an occasional pain in my side, but I'm sure it's just from riding my bicycle"). This type of presentation could easily result in a distorted description of what really is going on with your body. If the doctor does not have a clear picture of the problem, he might dismiss your symptom and miss an important diagnosis. We cannot overemphasize the fact that the way you actually present your symptoms to your doctor has a major impact on the diagnostic process. (See figures 11 and 12.)

A final suggestion for the interview is to be aware of the time limitations of an office visit. Whenever you present

---

Figure 11

Presentation of Symptoms (Heart Disease)

Misleading Presentation

"My chest feels funny for a short time when I'm at work. It's probably just the stress of my job."
The doctor may not pursue an investigation, thinking it's a trivial complaint.

Misleading Presentation

"Doctor, I've been getting indigestion lately. I think it's gas. Can you give me something for it?"
The doctor might try an antacid; she might consider getting abdominal X rays to check for an ulcer.

Clear Presentation

"I have chest pressure that feels like a fist tightening in the center of my chest. It began several weeks ago and lasts for a couple of minutes each time. I first noticed it after walking up a couple of flights of stairs at work. It felt better after I stopped to rest."
The doctor considers the possibility of heart disease and orders appropriate tests to check for this possibility.

---

several complaints or symptoms, the doctor must make the decision to ignore or investigate each one. You want to make sure the doctor understands your *primary concern* and is focusing his attention and time on evaluating your major symptoms. You should neither expect nor ask the doctor to make a detailed investigation and diagnosis

---

Figure 12

Presentation of Symptoms (Tension Headache)

Misleading Presentation

"I've been getting terrible headaches all the time. I never had anything like this before. I'm worried sick it's a tumor."
The doctor may suggest unneeded testing such as an expensive brain scan.

Misleading Presentation

"I'm getting bad headaches and wonder if my blood pressure is up."
The doctor checks blood pressure and finds it normal. Patient gets no explanation for cause of headache.

Clear Presentation

"For the last several months, I've been getting a bad headache. I'll get a tightening pain that begins in my neck and spreads to my temples. It occurs several times a week, usually in the afternoon, and lasts several hours. Do you think it could be a brain tumor?"
Symptoms are those of a muscular-tension headache, not the symptoms of a brain tumor. The doctor can reassure the patient without testing and try a simple pain reliever.

---

of a large number of unrelated complaints. If you do have several symptoms to present, let the doctor know what they are at first ("I have three things I would like to ask you about today"). This allows the doctor to have a sense of what will need to be done, and he can adjust his time accordingly. Otherwise, more serious concerns can get lost in the shuffle, and time better used in explanation is spent on numerous investigations.

In closing, we want to remind you again of the importance of the interview in reaching a diagnosis. It is the springboard or foundation of the diagnostic process, and your carefully considered input is critical. Use the outline we have provided for you and see the difference it makes during your next visit.

7

The Physical Examination

fter the interview is complete and the doctor has a clear picture of your symptoms, she considers the information available and proceeds to the next step of the diagnostic process, the physical examination. The doctor now looks for *signs* that correspond to the symptoms you have described. A sign is an abnormality found during the physical examination. For example, if the symptom you mention is an earache, the doctor would examine your ear and perhaps find a sign such as a red and swollen eardrum. Occasionally, a symptom will call for an examination of areas other than those that appear to be directly involved. For example, pain in your fingers could come from arthritis in your neck. The presence or absence of certain signs will determine the probability that the disease the physician has considered actually is present.

It is important for you to understand that signs are not always absolute indicators of the presence or absence of disease. After the interview, the doctor has at least one and maybe two or three ideas of what may be causing your symptoms. As she goes through the different parts of the physical examination, she is continually weighing the evidence provided by the signs that are present and the signs that are not. Although you may consider medicine an exact science, there is much judgment and "best guesswork" at various stages of the diagnostic process. The progression from symptom to sign to cause may be very simple, easily observed, and readily detected. On the other hand, there will be many instances when there is not a simple and obvious explanation, and the doctor must look for a cluster or group of symptoms, signs, and test results. In other words, the whole clinical picture must be presented before the pattern of data characteristic of a specific disease or condition can be identified.

Unlike the interview, the physical examination is pretty much in the hands of your doctor. Your role is limited, but it can be very helpful for you to know what to expect. The more familiar you are with the different procedures the doctor performs, the more comfortable and relaxed you will be during your visit. When you are more at ease, you may be better able to follow your doctor's instructions. Consequently, your doctor may obtain more precise data during the examination.

You can prepare for the physical examination in a few simple ways. For example, let your doctor know if you have noticed something on your body that seems different or if you have experienced discomfort in certain places. Don't assume she automatically will notice these changes. Also, you shouldn't be afraid to ask the doctor what she is looking for and why. Finally, the most important aspect of your role in the physical examination is cooperation.

The following sections of this chapter provide an account of the major components of a complete physical examination. Although you probably won't receive this type of exam when you visit the doctor for a specific complaint or concern, we think this information will be of interest to you. Specifically, knowing what the doctor generally looks for during a full physical examination will broaden your knowledge, help you to know what to expect during more focused exams, and, consequently, help you to feel more comfortable. This description is representative of an annual examination or checkup.

Vital Signs

Blood Pressure—Blood pressure is a measure of the pressure or force of the blood as it pushes against the inside lining of the arteries. In a sample pressure reading (130/80) the top number represents the *systolic* pressure, the pressure of the blood when the heart contracts. The bottom number represents the *diastolic* pressure, the pressure of the blood when the heart relaxes. Blood pressure is measured using a special cuff called a sphygmomanometer. The doctor essentially is checking for high blood pressure. If the pressure is too high, it can damage the arteries and cause blood clots to form.

Pulse Rate—The pulse rate is the measure of the number of times the heart beats per minute. Although the pulse rate is often quite low in athletes, a low rate can occasionally be a sign of some types of heart disease. An unusually high pulse rate can be associated with fever, an overactive thyroid, and anemia.

Respiratory Rate—The respiratory rate is the number of times a patient breathes per minute. The doctor checks to see if the rate is too high—which can indicate the possibility of certain types of lung disease.

Temperature—The doctor checks the body temperature. An elevated temperature could suggest infection. A slightly low temperature is not a sign of illness.

S k i n

The skin is examined from the hair on the head to the soles of the feet as the doctor looks for rashes, abnormal moles, and even changes of the hair and nails. Abnormalities usually represent a localized skin problem but could originate from an internal illness. For example, a facial rash could come from an allergy to makeup, but it could also be caused by lupus, a serious type of arthritis.

L y m p h   N o d e s

The lymph nodes are small glands composed of immune cells. They are scattered throughout the body and help defend against infection. Many of these glands are close enough to the surface of the body that the doctor can feel them when they enlarge. He examines the appropriate areas of the head, neck, arms, and groin. When you have a sore throat, you may feel enlarged lymph nodes in your neck. Persistent enlargement of the lymph nodes, however, can occur with more serious infections or even with certain tumors.

E y e s

Every part of the eye is examined. The doctor looks at the eyelid, the sclera (white area), the iris (pigmented area), and the pupil. Each part provides useful information. For example, a sclera that is abnormally yellow could represent liver disease. The doctor even looks inside the eye itself with a lighted magnifying lens called an ophthalmoscope. This allows him to examine the tissue layer at the back of the eye (the retina) and the blood vessels lying over it. Abnormalities here can occur with diseases as di-

verse as diabetes, hypertension, glaucoma, certain infections, and even brain tumors.

E a r s

The ears are inspected and evaluated for abnormalities of
the ear canal and ear drum. Swelling or redness can occur
with infection.

M o u t h

The doctor examines all aspects of the mouth including
the lips, tongue, cheeks, and throat, looking for early tumors. A thorough exam, however, might reveal additional
information. For example, an abnormally smooth tongue
could represent certain vitamin deficiencies.

N e c k

The neck is examined for signs of arthritis. In addition,
the doctor feels the thyroid gland, located at the base of
the neck. The thyroid gland secretes a hormone that con-
trols metabolism. The gland can become abnormally
large if it begins to malfunction. The doctor also feels for
nodules of the gland, which could represent a thyroid tumor. He examines the carotid arteries, the blood vessels
leading from the heart to the head, by feeling their pulse
and listening to them with a stethoscope. An abnormally
weak pulsation or a turbulent, flowing sound could represent a significant blockage.

L u n g s

The doctor examines the lungs by having you breathe in
and out while he listens with the stethoscope. He listens

for abnormal sounds that could indicate underlying lung disease, such as the soft wheezing of asthma, the crackling sound of pneumonia, or the diminished sounds of emphysema.

Heart

The heart is examined both while you are lying down and sitting up. When the patient is lying down the doctor first feels the left side of the chest for the pulsation of the heartbeat. The pulsation may be abnormal if the heart is enlarged. The doctor then listens with the stethoscope for abnormal sounds that could represent damage to the heart valves. Heart valves are firm leaflets of tissue that divide the heart into separate chambers. They act like doors opening and closing rhythmically to make certain the blood flows forward when the heart contracts. If any of them become diseased, the blood flow across them can become turbulent and produce an abnormal sound called a *murmur*. In addition, he listens for a regular rhythm to the heartbeat. An irregular rhythm may sometimes represent heart disease.

Abdomen

Although the abdomen contains the majority of the organs in the body, the doctor unfortunately can detect only a limited number of abnormalities by examining it. There are many organs that almost never produce any abnormal abdominal findings, such as the kidneys, the pancreas, the adrenals, and the bladder. Other organs may produce only vague, nonspecific findings such as tenderness. These organs include the stomach, gallbladder, and intestines. The doctor begins by using his stethoscope to listen for the sounds of the normally functioning intestines. He also listens over the large blood vessel deep within the abdomen called the aorta as well as over its branches. Abnormal sounds here could represent blockage. He then feels the entire abdomen for any tenderness that could be significant, and for masses that occasionally occur with large tumors. He specifically feels below the ribs on the right side for possible enlargement of the liver, below the ribs on the left for possible enlargement of the spleen, and deep within the midline for an abnormal swelling of a weakened aorta called an *aneurysm.*

Breasts

The doctor examines a woman's breasts in both the lying and sitting positions. He feels for abnormal masses and checks for abnormal secretions that could represent breast cancer. Men's breasts are examined for abnormal enlargement, which can occur with certain hormone abnormalities.

Back

The doctor examines the back for abnormal curvature, reduced flexibility, or abnormal tenderness.

Extremities

The joints are examined for evidence of arthritis by checking for abnormal swelling, tenderness, or diminished range of motion. The exam includes not only the larger joints such as the knees but also the smaller ones of the fingers. He checks the pulses of both wrists and both feet. A diminished or absent pulsation in an extremity can represent blockage of the associated artery. The shin of each leg is pressed to check for edema, an abnormal collection of fluid beneath the skin that can indicate disease of the kidneys, liver, or heart. Significant information can be gathered even from the fingernails. The nails can become abnormal with diseases as diverse as overactive thyroid to lung cancer.

Genitalia

The doctor examines the vagina, cervix, uterus, and ovaries in women; the testicles and penis in men. He looks for signs of infection, inflammation, or cancer.

Rectal

The rectum is examined for tumors or hemorrhoids. In men, the prostate is checked for abnormal enlargement or cancerous nodules.

Neurological

The doctor checks the reflexes, muscle strength, sensation, and coordination of the arms and legs. He compares one side with the other, knowing they should be equal, and notes any abnormal responses that could indicate an underlying disorder. Abnormal reflexes can occur with problems as varied as a previous stroke or an underactive thyroid gland. Sensation can be diminished by abnormalities as diverse as a pinched nerve, diabetes, or a vitamin deficiency.

We hope that this information will help you understand more about the nature of physical examinations and the potential role of selected parts of the exam in the diagnostic process. The extent to which your doctor examines you and where she examines you are related to the number or type of physical signs that would correspond to her suspected diagnosis. We remind you that there will be many times when a suspected diagnosis has *no* physical signs. For example, heart-artery disease, the blockage of arteries in the heart, which leads to heart attacks, has no signs a doctor could detect during the physical examination. Also, in the early stages of some diseases, physical findings may not yet be present. For example, some cancers do not produce abnormal findings on examination until late in their course.

Probably the most difficult part of a physical examination from the patient's perspective is wondering what is going on in the doctor's mind as she conducts the exam. As we've said, you can ask her to discuss her findings as she goes along. What is most important is the role the exam has played in the diagnostic process. Remember, the doctor has been looking for specific physical signs that will support a suspected diagnosis. While the absence of these signs does not definitely exclude the presumed diagnosis, their presence clearly strengthens the diagnostic case (see figure 13). The physical signs noted in the examination will be used in one of the following ways: (1) to support the doctor's original diagnosis; (2) to suggest to the doctor that she is on the right track and additional evaluation is needed; (3) to help rule out the original diagnosis. (In this last case the doctor can either continue to pursue the diagnosis through testing, or consider the presence of the illness highly unlikely.)

As she did after the interview section, the doctor will now stop, evaluate, and analyze the information she has received. If she feels satisfied that she knows what has caused your symptoms or is confident that she has ruled out any serious condition, she may stop the diagnostic process at this point. She may, however, feel that addi-

---

Figure 13
Roles of Physical Findings in a Diagnosis

Patient's complaint: weight loss. Doctor considers overactive thyroid or liver disease as possible causes. The following cases illustrate the possible role of physical findings.

Case 1: The doctor finds an *enlarged thyroid gland* and a *normal-sized liver.* The weight of evidence favors a diagnosis of an overactive thyroid.

Case 2: The doctor finds a *normal-sized thyroid gland* and *enlarged liver.* The weight of evidence favors a diagnosis of liver disease.

In Cases 1 and 2, the presence of physical finding does not prove a diagnosis; it only makes the diagnosis more likely.

Case 3: The doctor finds a normal-sized thyroid gland and normal-sized liver. The weight of evidence is unchanged. The doctor must still consider both possible diagnoses.

In Case 3, the absence of physical findings does not necessarily exclude a diagnosis; it may only make it less likely. In all three cases, the doctor may need to pursue further testing on both organs to exclude abnormality. The tests she decides to order first may be influenced by the above findings.

---

tional evidence is necessary either to support or rule out a specific diagnosis. If this is the case, there are several routes the doctor can pursue. These are addressed in the next chapter.

8

Diagnostic Tests

As you are now aware, when your doctor is ready to consider using diagnostic tests, he has already formulated a list of possible diagnoses. That is the only way he can know what tests to order. It is important that we keep tests and test results in the proper perspective. Tests can confirm a diagnosis, but they are rarely used to generate the diagnosis. Tests help to lessen the degree of uncertainty about the existence of a specific disease but frequently do not ensure the absolute absence or presence of the illness. In short, a test result is one more piece of the puzzle, one more bit of evidence. Patients sometimes overestimate the value of tests and assume they hold the key to a diagnosis. In fact, there will be times when you will be asked to accept a diagnosis or the exclusion of a diagnosis without the administration of a test. Your ability to follow what your doctor is doing will depend on your understanding of tests and their role in the diagnostic process. Just keep in mind that although tests can be extremely helpful and provide the doctor with clarification and specific information, they are rarely the focal point of the diagnostic procedure and seldom the sole means of identifying the cause of your symptoms.

Let's look now at a variety of both simple and complex diagnostic tests. We describe and give examples of some specific tests. We also provide you with general questions to ask your doctor both when you receive recommendations for testing and when you get the test results.

S i m p l e   Te s t s

As mentioned earlier, simple tests include blood and urine studies, the electrocardiogram, and simple X rays. Blood tests will be described more extensively later in this chapter.

A *urine analysis* screens for abnormal substances in the urine. For example, the presence of sugar could represent diabetes; protein could signify kidney disease. The urine specimen is also examined under the microscope for blood cells or bacteria that could represent infection, a kidney stone, or organ damage.

An *electrocardiogram* (EKG) provides information about electrical activity within the heart. The electrical activity is what stimulates the heart to beat. The EKG itself is a paper printout that shows recorded patterns representing this electrical activity. By interpreting these patterns, the doctor can sometimes diagnose heart damage; however, the printout can often appear completely normal in the presence of some types of significant heart disease.

A *simple X ray* is an X-ray photograph taken without using any special X-ray preparations or dyes. It can show a detailed image of bones but only vague outlines of the organs photographed. Pictures of the lungs, however, do show some of the internal structure in more detail because the lungs are filled with air. Simple X rays sometimes are not able to indicate very early abnormal changes and frequently cannot be used to identify the cause of the abnormalities they do detect. For example, a chest X ray might show an abnormal spot in the lungs, but without a biopsy, the doctor may not be able to tell if the spot represented a cancer or an infection.

Even though there are a few simple tests that will confirm whether a disease is present, such as the blood test for HIV, most simple tests only suggest that something is abnormal but do not uncover the precise diagnosis. A blood test that shows an elevated white blood cell count suggests the presence of an infection but gives no clue to where the infection might be located. Simple tests typically give information that lends weight to one of the diagnoses the doctor is considering but do not themselves constitute a diagnosis. Because these tests are generally low-risk, minimally invasive, and relatively inexpensive, the doctor is likely to order them without too much afterthought or concern.

We may have seemed to minimize the value of simple tests, but, as you will see in the following example, they can be very helpful in the diagnostic process. It is important, however, that you also realize their limitations. Because of the frequency of blood tests and the interest in them, we have chosen blood tests to illustrate the many uses of simple tests and the ways they can be used to support or exclude diagnoses.

B l o o d   T e s t s

There are literally over a thousand different blood tests. Some of these are specific tests for certain illnesses, and the doctor will order them only if he suspects the diagnosis corresponding to the positive or negative result he is looking for. The vast majority of illnesses, however, have no specific blood test to help the doctor diagnose them. Essentially, these tests inform the doctor that an abnormality may exist, without revealing the specific cause or source of the abnormality. For example, blood tests you may receive as part of a complete physical examination are designed to screen several major organ systems for abnormalities. One of the components of these routine blood studies is a blood creatinine. An abnormally high level alerts the physician to the possibility of kidney disease. The test itself does not indicate the cause of the damage. Another key problem is that a normal level of blood creatinine does *not* rule out the possibility of kidney disease.

Let's look in greater detail at the range of possible uses of blood tests. This information will be helpful as you try to understand the reasons your doctor may consider using them.

Blood tests can be used to diagnose specific abnormalities. As we've said, only a few blood tests can actually be used to provide definitive confirmation of a specific diagnosis. Two of these are the blood tests for HIV and sickle-cell anemia. In these cases, the doctor suspects the diagnosis and then orders the blood test for that specific disease to determine if the diagnosis is correct or not. We remind you that blood tests rarely can be used in this way, although it certainly would be easier to reach a diagnosis if there were a surefire blood test for every existing illness.

Blood tests can be used to support a suspected diagnosis. As indicated earlier, some blood tests can show that there is a change or elevation in certain blood substances. Although specific causes of the change are not revealed through the test, the doctor can use the information to strengthen his initial suspicion of a certain diagnosis. For example, if a patient complains of severe pain in the upper abdomen, one of the diagnoses to consider would be pancreatitis, an inflamed pancreas. Sometimes an inflamed pancreas produces an elevation of a blood component called amylase. If the results of a blood test did indicate elevated blood amylase, the doctor would have support for this diagnostic possibility.

Blood tests can be used to follow the progression or resolution of a disease. Some diseases produce abnormally elevated levels of certain components of the blood that return to normal when the disease resolves. The doctor can measure these components to determine whether the illness is improving or not. For example, hepatitis, an inflammation of the liver, damages liver cells. The liver damage causes the release of several substances called enzymes into the bloodstream. By measuring the level of these enzymes periodically, the doctor can monitor the status of this illness.

Blood tests can be used to get baseline measurements. As part of the initial evaluation of a new patient, the doctor frequently will order a routine series of blood tests. These studies can provide a variety of measurements, including levels of blood sugar and calcium, the red and white blood cell count, and assessments of liver and kidney function. When your doctor has baseline measurements he can refer back to these values later if a problem arises. By comparing current and baseline values, the doctor can determine whether changes have occurred and if the changes represent an abnormal development. The initial series of routine blood studies also can serve as a screen for certain conditions. Early diabetes, for example, could be uncovered by test results indicating elevated blood sugar.

Blood tests can provide new diagnostic information. Sometimes blood tests are used to search for clues when the patient interview and physical exam do not reveal any causes for the existing symptoms. If a doctor does not find anything abnormal during the physical exam in a patient complaining of chronic fatigue, he may order several blood tests. For example, he might check the blood for anemia to help him decide if a medical problem exists at all.

Blood tests can be used to evaluate levels of medication. Whenever administering medication it is important to ascertain the optimum dosage for the individual patient. This is particularly important with medications associated with potential risks or side effects or for those with a narrow range of effectiveness. For some of these medications, blood tests are available that determine the level of medication in the blood and therefore allow the doctor to optimize the dosage and avoid toxicity. For example, a blood test can be used to measure the level of digitalis in the blood. Digitalis is a drug used to treat certain types of heart disease. If the level is too low, it is ineffective; if the level is too high, it can be dangerous.

Blood tests can be used to monitor health maintenance. Certain blood tests provide important information that can help the patient preserve good health. For example, elevated blood cholesterol is a definite risk factor for subsequent heart disease and stroke. When elevated cholesterol is detected early and brought under control, these health problems can often be prevented.

Blood tests can determine side effects of certain medicines. Blood tests are also used to determine if some medications are having adverse effects on organs such as the liver or kidney. For example, isoniazid, a medicine used to treat tuberculosis, can sometimes damage the liver. If this problem is detected early with appropriate blood studies, the medication can be discontinued while the problem is still reversible.

In the section above, we have discussed the many uses of blood tests and the ways they can be helpful to your physician for multiple aspects of health care and maintenance. To give you a more complete understanding of how your doctor can use this information, we must also show you some of the difficulties of interpreting test results.

L i m i t a t i o n s   o f   B l o o d   T e s t s

Blood tests can lack sensitivity. A blood test may not detect slight amounts of the specific substance being tested. As a result of this lack of sensitivity, the test could be read as "normal" even though the disease being evaluated is present. For example, rheumatoid arthritis is associated with a specific diagnostic blood test called a *rheumatoid factor.* A small percentage of patients with rheumatoid arthritis test negative for this factor because it is present in a very small amount—too small for the blood test to register. If the doctor considers only the blood test and not the entire clinical picture, he will make an incorrect diagnosis.

Blood tests can lack specificity. A result that indicates one disease can test positive in other diseases as well. For example, the rheumatoid factor can sometimes be positive in lupus and scleroderma, two other types of arthritis. This lack of specificity makes it difficult to identify the disease the patient actually has without also considering other clinical factors.

Positive blood test results can lead to a false-positive diagnosis. A blood test can be abnormal even though no disease is present. This is called a *false-positive* test result. For example, a result that is slightly high or slightly low could represent a normal value for *you.* An illustration is the blood test for the liver substance called bilirubin. Although a positive test result can indicate liver disease, a number of people have slightly high levels of this substance, and an abnormal result may not represent disease for them. If the doctor considered only the elevated blood test in such cases, he might make the false-positive diagnosis of hepatitis.

One additional area to discuss is learning more about your test results. If your doctor has administered a blood test or a series of blood tests, you will want to discuss the results with him. If your tests come back as normal, and the doctor continues to express some concern, it is possible that he thinks the test may not have been sufficiently sensitive. He may want to retest at a later date or use another form of evaluation. As we've mentioned, this is an accepted limitation of some blood tests. If your test results come back with abnormal readings, it does not necessarily imply that you are ill. You should ask the following four questions when you discuss abnormal results.

1. What does this test measure?
2. What diseases could be represented by these results?
3. Is it possible that the test could be abnormal but still not represent disease? (A false positive)
4. What course of action do you recommend?

Complex Tests

If simple tests do not provide sufficient information, the doctor may decide to proceed with complex testing. Complex tests provide information of a more specific nature and are usually performed by a radiologist or other specialist. Frequently these tests can rule out a possible cause for your symptoms and sometimes can determine the actual cause of the problem. Because of the potential hazards of some tests for the patient, the doctor must have a high level of suspicion that a specific illness or injury exists to warrant using these tests.

Specialized X rays and scans detect changes in the size, shape, or structure of the organ examined. These tests are much more expensive than simple tests, sometimes cause discomfort, and occasionally carry a risk. A CAT scan of the head, a computerized X-ray study that gives an intricate image of the brain, is very costly. An intravenous pyelogram (IVP), a detailed kidney X ray, requires an injection of a specialized dye into the patient's vein. This can be moderately uncomfortable and occasionally causes a serious allergic reaction.

Another type of complex test (scoping) requires entry into the patient's body with scopes or tubes that allow the doctor to view an organ. These studies reveal abnormalities that are often too small to detect on an X ray. Scoping procedures, however, frequently are more expensive than complex X-ray studies and usually more uncomfortable. There is also a very slight risk of the procedure damaging the organ being studied. For example, a colonoscope—an instrument used to look at the colon—on rare occasion can puncture the organ.

Our final example of a complex test is the biopsy. A biopsy involves the removal of tissue in order to examine it under the microscope for abnormalities that do not show up in other tests. In a biopsy, tissue is removed either with a large needle or a surgical incision. Risks with this procedure include excessive bleeding, wound infection, and anesthetic complications.

Because of these potential problems and concerns, the doctor may choose to begin testing with a less sensitive test that poses fewer risks. In other words, the doctor may be willing to accept a little more uncertainty for a little less risk. If the less sensitive test detects an abnormality, he may make the diagnosis without additional testing. If the result is normal, the doctor must then decide whether he (and you) are willing to accept a low level of uncertainty or go on to the riskier test. As you might expect, the seriousness of the problem being assessed will have a great impact on the decision to do additional testing. See figures 14 and 15 for an illustration of these diagnostic considerations.

Figure 14

A forty-two-year-old housewife complains of lower backache. Pain has occurred for several days. The patient rearranged her living room a week ago. The physical exam is negative.

The Doctor's Decisions

The Doctor's Reasons

Does a urine exam. The result is negative.

Doctor thinks a urine infection is unlikely but a kidney infection could cause back pain. The test is inexpensive and painless.

The doctor does not order a back X ray at this time.

Even if the patient has arthritis, it would not influence the doctor's immediate treatment plan. If the pain persists, he can order an X ray later.

The doctor diagnoses low back strain, which he treats with bed rest and muscle relaxers. A follow-up appointment is scheduled for one to two weeks.

Testing and the Diagnostic Process

Throughout the diagnostic process, it is important that you recognize and understand your role as well as your

Figure 15

A fifty-year-old truck driver complains of seeing blood in his urine yesterday. He has had no pain. The physical exam shows nothing abnormal.

The Doctor's Decisions	*The Doctor's Reasons*
The doctor does a urine exam. The results show red blood cells in the specimen.	The test confirms that the patient does have blood in his urine. The cause is still unknown.
The doctor orders an IVP.* The test is negative.	A kidney tumor or stone now is unlikely. A bladder stone or tumor, however, often does not show up on an IVP.
The doctor orders a cystoscopy.**	Even though the cystoscopy is uncomfortable, expensive, and has a slight risk, the physician feels the potential for serious disease is significant enough to warrant further testing.
The cystoscopy shows a small bladder tumor.	

*An X-ray test. A dye is injected into the patient's vein and is filtered by the kidneys. Both the kidneys and the bladder will then show up when x-rayed.

**The doctor passes a short, narrow fiberoptic tube into the bladder. Because of fiberoptics, the doctor can actually see the bladder lining.

physician's role. By the time the testing phase is reached, the doctor already has definite ideas about what is causing your symptoms. His intention is to confirm or reject the diagnoses he is considering. What is your role at this stage? Because of the many uses as well as limitations of tests, it is critical that you know what questions to ask your doctor and when to ask them. As you probably realize, even when the doctor presents you with a series of alternatives, he still recommends the one he feels is best. Most of us follow the doctor's advice because we feel that his experience, knowledge, and professional judgment support his recommendations. Sometimes there will be several viable options, however, and it is important for you to understand them and why the doctor suggests one over another. Usually, his suggestions are based on the nature of the suspected illness. Your doctor may strongly recommend testing if he is considering a serious illness or one that could be clearly identified through a diagnostic test. For less significant possibilities, he may feel further testing is optional or not immediately critical (see figure 16).

When testing is recommended, your participation is required. Although the test itself may not require your help, agreeing to the test and showing up are both up to you. No test can be administered without your consent. Sometimes you may be afraid to follow up on recommended testing because of your fear of a particular disease. You may not see the need for testing, as in the case of a single occurrence of a symptom. Whether your reason is discomfort, fear, cost, or indifference, the result of not having necessary testing could be the same—a missed diagnosis. Therefore, we believe that an active search for answers to questions related to testing is important for your information, peace of mind, and confidence in the evaluation. The following questions will help you learn more about any test your doctor recommends.

Figure 16

A thirty-eight-year-old teacher complains of abdominal burning. Pain has occurred intermittently for several weeks. The patient has found that antacids relieve the pain. The physical exam shows nothing abnormal.

The Doctor's Decisions

The doctor orders an upper GI,* which is negative.

The doctor decides not to do further testing and elects not to do an endoscopy.**

The doctor diagnoses gastritis.*** He treats it for one month with a pill that eliminates stomach acid secretion. A follow-up visit is scheduled in two weeks. The work-up may be pursued if pain persists.

The Doctor's Reasons

The doctor looks for a possible ulcer with this test. The discomfort and risk of this test are minimal. He would like a definite diagnosis if it can be made easily.

The doctor knows that an upper GI fails to detect an ulcer 20 percent of the time when one is present. Still he knows there is an 80 percent chance that his patient does not have an ulcer.

The doctor feels that the need to be certain about the presence of an ulcer does not warrant the discomfort or expense of endoscopy. The medication should relieve the patient's pain and should heal an ulcer if one exists.

*The patient drinks a chalky-tasting liquid called barium that outlines the stomach and small intestine when x-rayed.

**The doctor passes a long fiberoptic tube down the patient's esophagus into the stomach. Because of fiberoptics, the doctor can actually see the stomach lining.

***Irritation to the stomach from excess acid but not enough to cause actual ulceration.

1. What will this test show you? Are there others that would give similar information?
2. How is the test done? Is it uncomfortable?
3. Are there any risks (e.g., radiation, possible allergic reactions, anesthesia)?
4. If the test results are negative (normal), could I still have the problem or disease?
5. Will this be the only test necessary or will you need others to make the diagnosis? (See figure 17.)

What if your doctor is unsure of the precise cause of your condition but wants to "wait and see" instead of recommending further testing? He may feel that the symptoms do not suggest anything significant and prefer to observe you for several weeks before doing any further evaluation. He suspects the symptoms will just go away and wants to save you the discomfort and expense of unnecessary tests. Your doctor may even suggest that your symptom be left untreated, hoping to gain information that could be masked by medication. For example, it would be difficult to tell if your fever were getting higher if you were taking aspirin on a regular basis. He reasons that even if something is abnormal and your symptoms do persist, the short delay will not affect you adversely. In these circumstances, it is always best for you to understand his reasoning and feel comfortable with his advice. Remember that the decision to delay further evaluation could arise at any stage of the diagnostic process. Your doctor's responses to the following three simple questions should help you feel less worried during the period of observation.

1. Why do you prefer waiting to testing?
2. What significant diseases have you excluded?
3. What symptoms should I look out for that could suggest complications?

Figure 17

Sonogram of the Gallbladder

Patient: "What will this test show you? Are there others that would give similar information?"

Doctor: "The test will show whether or not you have stones in your gallbladder. There is another test where you take several iodine pills that cause the gallbladder to show up when x-rayed. It is no more sensitive than a sonogram and carries a risk of an allergic reaction and radiation exposure."

Patient: "How is the test done? Is it uncomfortable?"

Doctor: "A sonogram is a test that uses sound waves to image the organ. A microphone is placed on the abdomen that both produces the sound waves and detects the echo. It is not uncomfortable at all."

Patient: "Are there any risks?"

Doctor: "There are no risks."

Patient: "If the test results are negative, could I still have the problem?"

Doctor: "It is very unlikely that gallstones are present if this test is negative. Occasionally, if the stones are very small, they won't show up and the test would be interpreted as normal."

Patient: "Will this be the only test necessary or will you need others to make the diagnosis?"

Doctor: "This is the only test we will need to do to check your gallbladder. If it shows gallstones, we will have to talk about possible surgery. If it doesn't, I feel it is extremely unlikely your pain is coming from your gallbladder. We may then have to test for other possible causes."

We hope this information helps you better understand the role of tests in the diagnostic process and allows you to feel more comfortable if you must undergo testing in the future. When test results indicate an abnormality, the doctor may have a confirmed diagnosis. He may be confident that the disease he suspects is present. If test results are normal, he may be equally confident that the disease is *not* present.

As we've stressed, the test result is just one part of the entire clinical picture. It usually helps only to assure the doctor that he has made the correct diagnosis. In many cases the doctor cannot rely solely on a test to identify completely or reject absolutely the presence of disease. Many tests are not 100 percent sensitive and don't always uncover the abnormality they were designed to detect. For example, as discussed in figure 17, an upper GI fails to detect an ulcer 20 percent of the time when it is actually present. Other tests may sometimes suggest an abnormal finding when disease is not actually present. An exercise stress test, for example, is designed to detect heart-artery disease. It is similar to an EKG, but the recording is done while the patient is exercising. Unfortunately, the test can look abnormal in 20 percent to 30 percent of patients with *normal* heart arteries. The bottom line is that we don't want you to expect a definitive answer from your doctor simply because you took a test. The entire diagnostic picture, coupled with your doctor's professional judgment, is the route to the answer, although not always the final one. The fact that there usually is some degree of uncertainty in a medical diagnosis is one of the most difficult concepts to accept, for both patients and physicians.

In the next chapter, we will summarize the results of the diagnostic process and look at ways to understand your illness and its treatment. We also discuss what to consider if no diagnosis is made. Once again, there are many opportunities for you to participate and ask questions. We will continue to explore the ways you can work with your doctor to feel comfortable with the results and maximize the effectiveness of subsequent interventions.

9

Concluding the Diagnostic Process

In the previous chapters, we have reviewed the diagnostic process and its three components: the interview, the physical examination, and the diagnostic tests. At any point in this process your doctor may arrive at a conclusion about the cause of your symptoms. This chapter will be devoted to what happens when your doctor reaches a decision. We will consider not only possible conclusions from a diagnostic perspective but also how these conclusions may influence your feelings about what your doctor says and recommends. Your participation relating to possible courses of action will be a major focus of the chapter.

A Diagnosis Is Made

One conclusion that can result from the diagnostic process is the diagnosis of a specific cause for your symptoms. The doctor determines that a certain disease, condition, or injury has produced the pain or discomfort that brought you to her office in the first place. She has sifted through all the evidence you have provided and all she has observed, and one condition has surfaced as the likely cause. Now that you know the diagnosis, how will you react? What questions will you have? What if you aren't certain her diagnosis is correct?

Although there are several possible answers to these questions, they are all important considerations. Let's look at some possible responses.

Reactions to a Diagnosis

Although most people are usually relieved to get a diagnosis—to know why they feel the way they do—the diagnosis of a serious illness can be stressful and scary. The reactions to a diagnosis, therefore, can range from relief when it is nothing serious to fear or panic when it is. If you are confident of your doctor's diagnosis, even if it is something you don't want to hear, the next step is to learn about your illness. Whether the diagnosis is a minor ailment or a serious disease, understanding your illness is critical. Issues such as the best course of treatment, compliance with your doctor's recommendations, and assuring the maximum potential for future good health all depend on the degree to which you understand your illness and its implications for your well-being and lifestyle.

Some patients complain that their problems or treatments are not explained adequately by their doctors. You can alleviate the situation by asking your doctor to outline the basic points of the illness, explain its significance to your health, and discuss with you how she will treat it. By asking the questions below, you will be assured of a fuller understanding of your illness.

Questions to Ask About Your Diagnosis

1. *Why or how did I get this illness?* Your doctor should outline the reasons you have become ill and explain the significance to your health. You need to learn if it is contagious so that you can avoid giving it to others (for example, hepatitis, tuberculosis).

2. *Can this disease progress? What organs might become involved?* It is important to learn the prognosis for your illness. Will it be short-lived and respond to treatment or chronic and possibly progressive? If it is chronic, you will want to learn what to expect in the future.

3. *Are there any changes I can make that will improve the outcome?* It is very important to learn if life-style changes, such as weight loss or exercise, can improve the outlook of your illness or possibly allow it to go away. For example, sometimes diabetes can be reversed with weight loss and dietary changes. Other illnesses that aren't necessarily chronic are less likely to recur with certain changes. For example, bronchitis is much less likely to recur if a patient stops smoking.

4. *What effect will medications have on my illness and how long will I need to take them?* If the doctor prescribes medication, you need to learn whether it will cure the illness, slow its progression, or only alleviate the symptoms. It's also imperative that you know how long treatment is required. For an acute illness such as pneumonia, two weeks of antibiotics are usually adequate to cure it, whereas for chronic problems such as high blood pressure, therapy is usually lifelong.

5. *How can I become more educated about my illness?* The answers to the previous questions will give you a good understanding of your illness. For many chronic illnesses, however, there are many details you need to

learn that cannot be adequately described in a fifteen-minute office visit. Diabetes, for example, can have a major impact on many facets of a patient's life. To make the appropriate commitment for adequate treatment, a patient must fully understand it. Your doctor should be able to refer you to different sources from which you can get additional, understandable information.

Sometimes the doctor explains the situation using technical medical terms that are unfamiliar. It is imperative that you understand exactly what your doctor tells you. If you don't say anything or ask any questions, she will assume you understand what she is saying. This is not the time to feel shy or foolish about asking your doctor to repeat her explanation or to explain the situation using simpler terms. Your comprehension is what counts. It may help to take notes while your doctor is talking. In fact, to be certain that what you heard is actually what was said, it's best to repeat back her explanation or advice. Sometimes it may help if you ask the doctor to draw a picture or diagram for you.

The time you actually receive the diagnosis might not be the best time for you to take in all of the information your doctor gives you. This is particularly true if you have received the diagnosis of a serious illness. You may be upset, and many things will be going through your mind at once. In such circumstances, you might want to ask your doctor if you could call her or set up an office visit at a later time to discuss the details of your illness.

Questioning the Diagnosis

There could be an occasion when you receive a diagnosis but question its accuracy. There are many possible reasons you might feel this way. Maybe you've read something that seems to contradict your doctor's conclusion. Perhaps you have a history of a certain disease in your family and feel certain this is what you have. You may feel that your doctor was not thorough enough in his questioning, examination, or testing procedures. If you are concerned, ask your doctor how she arrived at the diagnosis. She should explain the process she used to rule out other potential causes and arrive at the one she has identified. If you have used the previous chapters to guide you through your office visits and have asked the recommended questions, you have the information you need to help you understand the diagnostic process and your doctor's explanation. If you are not satisfied with your doctor's explanation, or you think she has prematurely dismissed certain possibilities, then other options are available. One of these is to ask about the possibility of additional testing; another is to ask to see another physician who specializes in the area of your illness (your doctor may recommend this anyway).

Before you look at alternatives, however, it is best to examine the reasons for your unhappiness. You may be upset with the diagnosis even though you suspect it may be accurate. For example, a patient who drinks too much may not want to hear that his abdominal pain comes from excess alcohol. In the case of a serious illness, you may have trouble believing it is true even though you feel you have a good doctor. In these instances, discuss the situation with your doctor. She probably has other patients who have had similar difficulty accepting or believing that they have a certain problem and can recommend ways to help you feel secure in the diagnosis. Your physician knows you must accept your illness before you will participate and cooperate in appropriate treatment. It will be easier for both of you and any other doctor you might see if you all work together to arrive at the best course of action.

A Diagnosis Is Not Made

The second possible result of the diagnostic process is that no actual diagnosis is made. The doctor may feel that it is not necessary to pursue a definite diagnosis. She is confident that the possibilities are not significant problems and, as important, that a diagnosis would not affect the course of treatment. For instance, certain types of muscle pain may have several different causes, but the same treatment would be applied regardless of how or why the muscle was injured. A specific diagnosis, therefore, would not be required for appropriate treatment.

There will be other times when the doctor feels she has ruled out all possible serious diseases or abnormalities that could be responsible for your symptoms. This decision is not unusual (many symptoms seem to have no identifiable cause) and represents a valid and valuable diagnostic conclusion. Some of us may take the results and run, relieved that there is no evidence that something serious is wrong. Others, however, may be concerned about the lack of a specific diagnosis. They might think the doctor hasn't recognized their concern about the symptoms or hasn't taken their complaints seriously. Some patients actually want the doctor to find something wrong. For example, an overweight, overworked executive might prefer being told his chronic fatigue is due to a hormone imbalance rather than his frenzied life-style. Then it would be the doctor's responsibility to deal with the problem rather than his own.

How should you respond to the lack of a diagnosis? What are the questions to ask that will help you feel more comfortable with your doctor's conclusion? Regardless of the degree to which you are satisfied with your doctor's conclusions, the following questions will help to satisfy your concerns.

Questions to Ask About the Absence of a Diagnosis

1. *What significant illnesses have you ruled out?* As always, you will want to learn what possible causes your doctor considered and how she excluded them. This will be particularly helpful if you have been harboring a concern about a specific illness or have felt that your symptoms were similar to those of someone you know who had a particular illness. If your doctor doesn't mention an illness you are particularly worried about, ask her.

2. *Could I still have anything serious? Are there other symptoms I should look for?* You want to explore with your doctor the possibility that your symptoms might represent an illness that cannot yet be diagnosed—perhaps the illness is in too early a stage, or the present symptoms are too vague. You will want to know if there are other symptoms that could later cause her to change her opinion.

3. *Are there any other tests that could give you more information? If so, why haven't you wanted to use them?* As we discussed in the chapter on diagnostic tests, there will be times when your doctor makes choices about what tests she will recommend. If you have not already discussed these test choices with her, ask her to explain her rationale.

4. *Do you think a specialist could be helpful?* You will want to know if your doctor feels that another doctor with expertise in a particular area would be able to provide additional diagnostic information. Your doctor herself might recommend a specialist if she still has doubts about her conclusions. If she does not, and you still want to explore the possibility, discuss it with her. Chances are, if she has not already suggested a specialist she doesn't feel it is necessary, but that

doesn't mean she won't consider it. If you decide to seek a consultation on your own, it is still best to ask your doctor about the type of specialist you should see and the name of someone she would recommend. Discuss what kind of testing a specialist is likely to do. Ask what kind of information he could give that might differ from what your doctor already has given you. Always work with your doctor—she can give the specialist your previous test results so you can avoid unnecessary repeat testing. If the specialist has your complete medical profile it will save you both time and money.

What should you do if you feel the doctor simply hasn't investigated thoroughly or isn't knowledgeable enough to identify the real problem? If you are concerned about the thoroughness or quality of your doctor's procedures, it is important for you to know why. Is it more than the absence of a diagnosis that has made you think that your doctor is less than competent? Has the doctor previously been unresponsive to your input, ignored your request for explanations, or refused to take your concerns seriously? Do you feel the need to surreptitiously "check up" on her abilities? If your answer to any of these questions is yes, then you don't have the type of positive interaction with your doctor necessary to develop trust and confidence in her diagnostic abilities. In this case, you need to discuss the situation with your doctor and if you are not satisfied with the ensuing relationship you should seek a doctor who you feel is more responsive to your needs.

After the diagnostic process is concluded, there is still one more decision that needs to be made—how to treat the illness. In the next chapter, we discuss the two major types of treatment: medication and surgery.

10

Treating the Illness

W hether or not you received a diagnosis, you came to the doctor's office because you were experiencing symptoms that were causing you pain, discomfort, or concern. The final major decisions made by your doctor are when and how to treat your symptoms and/or your illness.

There will be times when the doctor simply doesn't believe that any treatment is necessary. Some patients expect a prescription for medication when they come to the doctor. They may even have a specific medication in mind, such as penicillin for a cold. (Penicillin, however, would not help a cold because it is ineffective against the cold virus.) For patients who expect a prescription, medication may represent more than treatment of an illness. It can serve as proof that their problem is real and that the doctor can do something to cure it. If the doctor doesn't prescribe anything, does it mean the visit wasn't needed or he hasn't uncovered the true problem? No. The doctor just feels the problem doesn't require theatment. If you are ever concerned about the lack of a prescription, you should ask your doctor to explain the medical reasons behind his decision.

Occasionally your doctor uses treatment to confirm a diagnosis. If the condition he suspects is known to improve with a specific medication, the doctor can prescribe it and see how you respond. If your symptoms are eliminated or greatly reduced, he may conclude that the diagnosis was correct. For example, if you have been experiencing recurrent, severe, throbbing headaches, the doctor may suspect you are having migraine headaches. He prescribes propranolol, a medication that sometimes helps prevent them. If your headaches improve significantly, this supports his initial diagnosis. If they don't, then he must consider other possibilities. This type of treatment is referred to as a *therapeutic trial*. A specific therapy or treatment is given for a trial period to see if it improves your symptoms. If it does, the doctor can use that information to confirm a diagnosis.

In most instances, of course, treatment is given after the diagnosis has already been made. There are many types of treatment you might receive from your doctor or from other physicians. The most common form of treatment is medication.

Medication — Questions to Ask

Except for antibiotics, most medications do *not* cure illness. Usually they are given to relieve the discomfort of your symptoms or to slow the progression of an illness. It is important for you to know the difference. If the medication is to ease discomfort, you can decide whether the pain is severe enough to require relief. If the medication is to slow the progression of your illness, you will better understand why it is important for you to take it regularly. Always ask the following questions:

1. *Why am I taking this medication?* Learn whether the

purpose of the medication is to treat your illness or just to lessen your discomfort. For example, most medications given for arthritis reduce pain and inflammation but do not slow down damage to the joints. On the other hand, blood pressure medication actually lessens the likelihood of damage to blood vessels and, therefore, can prevent subsequent stroke or heart disease.

2. *How will I know it is working?* You need to know how you can monitor the effectiveness of the medication you take. If your medication is to treat an acute illness, such as antibiotics for a urinary infection, learn how long it will take before you begin to feel better. If it is for a chronic illness, such as arthritis, learn if you should expect complete resolution of the pain or only partial relief. For illnesses that produce no symptoms, such as high blood pressure, treatment will not affect how you feel. The only way to determine the medication's effectiveness is to monitor the blood pressure periodically.

3. *Is there any other form of treatment available besides this medication?* Your doctor usually has a reason for his choice of medication to treat your illness or symptom. Sometimes there are several alternatives. For example, there are many different medications available to treat high blood pressure. They differ in cost, dosing schedule, and possible side effects. Your doctor should discuss these differences with you when you inquire about them.

4. *Are there any risks or side effects?* Most medications are extremely safe. Some, however, carry a slight risk of a toxic or allergic reaction. For example, some antibiotics occasionally cause liver or kidney damage. You will want to learn these possibilities beforehand. Most side effects are not dangerous or damaging to the body. They are only annoying symptoms produced by the

medication. Many sinus medications, for example, cause drowsiness. You won't worry as much about certain symptoms if you know they are only insignificant side effects. You can then let the doctor know if they are uncomfortable enough to require changing medication.

5. *How long will I need to take this medication and will this need be reevaluated periodically?* Some illnesses require only a week or two of treatment; others must be treated for many years. Medication to treat high blood pressure or diabetes, for example, usually must be taken for life. Sometimes, however, proper diet or weight loss will improve these conditions and your doctor may then be able to reconsider the need for continued treatment.

Although you should be given specific instructions with every type of medication you receive, there are certain universal rules to remember when taking prescription drugs. The following recommendations are extremely important and could be critical to your health.

Stopping medication: Always check with your doctor before altering the schedule or dose of medication prescribed. If you think a medication is making you feel ill, discuss it with your doctor before stopping it on your own. It can be dangerous to discontinue some medicines abruptly. For example, stopping certain blood pressure medications can cause a sudden, severe elevation in blood pressure. Also, stopping antibiotics because you feel better can result in only partial treatment and subsequent recurrence of your infection.

Other prescriptions: Never use an old prescription for a treatment without first consulting your doctor. You may only partially treat your problem by not taking the medication long enough or by using an incorrect dosage. In addition, some old medicines become toxic over time;

others become ineffective. For the same reasons, never experiment with someone else's medication.

Knowing your medications: It is important to be familiar with all of the medications you are taking. If you take several, keep a card in your wallet or purse listing their names, when prescribed, their dosages, and the illness each treats. Update the list any time your doctor makes a change. It's also a good idea to record any medicine that has previously produced a significant side effect or drug allergy (see figure 18). Your doctor can compare his list of medicines with yours and learn whether you take each one correctly. This also allows you to review periodically your doctor's list to double-check its accuracy. In addition, if you must see another doctor for an emergency, his detailed knowledge of your medicines may provide information crucial to your care.

Surgery — Questions to Ask

Unlike most medications, surgery can often eliminate the problem for which it is recommended. For example, if a

---

Figure 18
Medication Chart

Date Begun	Name	Dose	Frequency	Treats
9/6/93	Tenormin	50 mg.	once a day	high blood pressure
10/8/93	HCTZ	25 mg.	once a day	high blood pressure
10/8/93	K-Lor	20 meq.	twice a day	potassium replacement
1/4/94	Allopurinol	300 mg.	once a day	gout

Allergic to penicillin—causes rash

patient has recurrent abdominal pain from gallstones, removal of the gallbladder cures the condition. On the other hand, surgery is a more drastic intervention than other treatments and, consequently, requires greater participation on your part to feel comfortable with the doctor's advice. It is important to know what to expect from surgery—when it is needed to cure your condition and when it is recommended only as the best alternative to alleviate your symptoms. Below we list important questions to ask before considering surgery. It is best to discuss these questions with your own doctor as well as with the surgeon he suggests.

1. *Why do you recommend surgery and is there a danger to my health if I don't have it?* Sometimes the doctor advises surgery to alleviate painful symptoms that aren't actually a danger to your health. For example, with advancing age, some women develop an abnormal enlargement of the uterus from benign growths called fibroids. The enlarged uterus can cause recurrent lower abdominal pain but isn't usually detrimental to good health. The patient should decide if the discomfort is severe enough to warrant surgery.

2. *Do I need surgery now or could it wait?* Some conditions require an operation as soon as possible. This is obviously true of life-threatening emergencies such as a ruptured appendix, and it is true for conditions in which a delay might prevent a favorable outcome, such as the removal of a malignant tumor. On the other hand, some conditions will improve with surgery but are unlikely to worsen with a short delay. A hernia is an example of a condition of this type.

3. *What are the risks of this operation and does my medical condition or age increase the normal risks?* Even minor surgery poses a slight risk, such as excessive bleeding or wound infection. Certain chronic condi-

tions—diabetes or heart disease, for example—increase the risk of more serious complications. Very young or elderly people may run additional risks. It is important to be fully aware of these possibilities before you agree to surgery.

4. *Do doctors differ in their opinions about the need for surgery to treat my problem?* Sometimes doctors have different opinions about the relative value of surgery for certain conditions. Unique aspects of your case might cause some doctors to choose different approaches to treatment. If both your own doctor and a surgeon believe that surgery is indicated, you can usually feel comfortable with the decision. Many patients still prefer the opinion of a second surgeon. In fact, some insurance companies require a second surgical opinion before proposed nonemergency surgery.

5. *Are there any new or experimental therapies for my condition not yet available in our community?* As we all know, the rapidity of advances in modern medicine is startling. Some conditions that formerly required an operation can now be treated without one. For example, a machine has been introduced recently that destroys kidney stones with high-frequency sound waves. Surgery is no longer the only means to treat this condition. Some of the newest therapies or technologies may not be available in every hospital. If you learn that your problem can be managed without surgery at another site, you can then decide if you want to go there for treatment.

Other Treatments

Other forms of treatment include life-style changes such as stopping smoking, drinking less alcohol, increasing exercise, and eating a more healthful diet. As the saying

goes, "It's easier said than done," but if you fully understand why your doctor feels you need to make any of
these important changes, you are much more likely to
make the necessary commitment. (Additional types of
treatment, such as radiation therapy and chemotherapy,
are beyond the scope of this book.)

11

Consulting a
Specialist

Your primary-care doctor monitors your health and provides you with continuing medical care. There are times, however, when your doctor will seek the opinion of a specialist to help with a diagnosis or to perform a specific procedure. It is important, therefore, that you understand the role of the specialist in your health care. In this chapter we define the term *specialist* and show you how to interact with a specialist effectively. We will focus on why you or your doctor might consider it important for you to see one. Finally, we will review the visit itself.

A specialist is a doctor whose focus is one specific area or system of the body. After completing requirements for general medicine or surgery, a physician may choose to continue with several years of additional training to gain expertise in a specialty area. She also learns to perform and interpret specific procedures. There are specialists in both the medical and surgical branches of medicine; often there are medical and surgical specialists for the same organ system. The medical specialist deals primarily with diagnosis and treatment, often using sophisticated tests and procedures. The surgical specialist also employs diagnostic procedures, but her major focus is performing operations. For example, the medical specialist dealing with problems of the heart and circulatory system is a cardiologist; the surgical specialist is a cardiac surgeon. The medical specialist who diagnoses and treats diseases that affect kidney function is a nephrologist; the surgical specialist who performs surgery and other invasive procedures on the bladder and kidneys is a urologist.

There are specialists for all of the different organ systems, and in some other areas as well. There are 13 specialty areas in medicine, and 9 specialty areas in surgery. In the Glossary we present a list of the many types of specialists and provide a brief description of each of them. Although the number may be somewhat overwhelming, your primary-care physician should help you in selecting the appropriate one.

There are two possible reasons for seeing a specialist— either your doctor wants a referral or you do. Although we strongly suggest that you make use of your physician's knowledge and opinion when consulting a specialist, we recognize that this does not always happen.

Patient Self-referral

A number of people who don't have a primary-care doctor choose their own specialist when a problem arises. This requires the individual to identify the area of abnormality and then select the correct corresponding specialist. This approach has many potential drawbacks, including the possibility of selecting the wrong type of doctor. For example, after feeling persistent chest pain, a patient might go straight to the cardiologist. Many expensive tests later, he learns that the source of pain is not the heart, and that the appropriate specialist would have been a gastroenter-ologist because the pain was actually caused by an ulcer. Remember that the specialist focuses on specific and often complex diagnostic procedures. If you present symptoms to her, she is bound by both professional and legal accountability to investigate the problems in detail to rule out disease in her area. This can be time-consuming, quite expensive, and occasionally unnecessary. Frequently, the problem could have been evaluated by a primary-care doctor, often with less extensive testing.

Other individuals who already have a primary-care doctor may choose to go to a specialist on their own because they don't fully trust their primary-care doctor or don't want to hurt his feelings. As a result, the specialist is required to start from scratch because he may be unaware of testing that has already been done. The patient also does not benefit from the opinion of his own doctor about the quality of the specialist chosen. Of course, the major problem in these instances is the relationship between the patient and the primary-care doctor. If a patient trusts his primary-care physician and can trust his decisions, he can feel more confident that the specialist chosen will be conscientious and competent.

Physician Referrals

You usually will see a specialist on the advice of your physician. When the referral is made by your physician, you can be more comfortable that an appropriate and qualified specialist has been selected. There are a variety of reasons for referral. Some are based on the need for more medical knowledge, or evaluation; others originate because of the patient's concerns or feelings. Below we outline the reasons your physician may initiate a referral.

1. He may want a certain procedure or test conducted to

help make a diagnosis or rule out a serious condition. For example, he might refer a patient with blood in the urine to a urologist for diagnostic testing to determine its cause.

2. Your doctor may want a second opinion about the significance of a worrisome symptom or an abnormal physical finding. For example, a patient with chest pain may be referred to a cardiologist to help decide if further tests are indicated. A patient with a breast lump might be sent to a surgeon to help determine if a biopsy should be done.

3. Your doctor may encounter a diagnostic dilemma: a situation in which something is clearly wrong (for example, an unexplained, rapid thirty-pound weight loss), but the doctor cannot determine the cause. In such cases, the patient may be referred to a specialist for further evaluation.

4. Your illness requires sophisticated treatment or has not responded to the treatment your doctor has already prescribed. For example, chemotherapy is almost always given by an oncologist, a cancer specialist.

5. Finally, your primary-care doctor may recommend you to a surgical specialist to determine the need for an operation and, if necessary, to perform surgery. A patient with cataracts would be referred to an ophthalmologist for eye surgery.

Sometimes your physician makes a referral because you've asked for one. Your doctor should be willing to recommend an appropriate specialist to address any of your concerns. Here are several reasons a patient may ask for a specialist consultation:

1. The primary care doctor may not be able to identify the cause of a persistent symptom that is worrisome to the patient, such as fatigue or lethargy. The patient

may ask the doctor for a referral to a specialist to see if a diagnosis has been missed.

2. Sometimes the patient does not agree with or does not want to accept his doctor's diagnosis (particularly an unpleasant one). He may then ask for a consultation with a specialist to confirm the original diagnosis.

3. A patient's problem may be diagnosed but is not responding to the prescribed treatment. The patient may ask to see a specialist to determine if alternative treatments are available.

Although these reasons represent concern, and to some extent dissatisfaction with the current care, a good doctor will understand your concern and your desire to have a specialist consult on the condition. In fact, she may be just as frustrated as you are if you are not responding to a specific treatment. By letting your doctor make the referral, you increase the likelihood that your visit with the specialist will be as helpful to you as possible.

How to Choose a Specialist

Earlier we presented a number of ways to select a primary-care doctor. The same process applies when choosing a specialist. It is important to realize, however, that the *best* way to select a specialist is through the recommendation of your primary-care doctor, who will be in a position to judge the technical competence and diagnostic skills of the specialist. The technical expertise of a specialist is of particular importance, and unless you will be seeing her for a long time, expertise is much more critical here than personal characteristics. If you are willing to travel to get a possibly higher level of expertise, let your doctor know—otherwise he is likely to make his recommendation based on local physicians.

There are questions you can ask your doctor about the

specialist he recommends to gain more information and to feel more confident about the referral. It is a good idea to ask why your doctor has recommended this particular person and to ask him to identify what he sees as the strengths and weaknesses of this specialist. You also should ask your doctor if he has referred other patients to this specialist and ask what their reactions were. You might even ask for the names of two specialists and your doctor's opinions about each of them. By asking questions like these, you can have a good idea of why your doctor has selected this specialist before making your appointment, and you will be more likely to feel comfortable with this particular physician.

Visiting the Specialist

Before the appointment with the specialist, you and your doctor should discuss the upcoming visit. It is important you understand fully what will occur in the specialist's office. Questions to ask your doctor include:

1. What are the reasons for this referral?
2. What tests or procedures is the specialist likely to do during my visit?
3. Whom should I contact about test results?
4. What other tests or procedures might the specialist recommend? Should I contact you before these are done?

When these questions are answered, you will have a good idea of what the specialist should do and what she might suggest. You also want to make sure the specialist has all the necessary information about your case. This should include the reason for the referral, your relevant past medical problems, and the results of tests already performed. This will prevent any overlap in procedures or tests that have been done previously. In figure 19 we provide a form that will ensure that all of this is done. Copy this form, and ask your doctor to fill it out and send it to the specialist before your visit. In addition, you should bring a list of your medications and how they are taken. This will help the specialist make knowledgeable decisions if she decides to administer treatment, or if she notices a particular symptom that may be a side effect of medication.

Because both the primary-care physician and the specialist are doctors and have similar goals, the approaches and techniques we suggested you use during the office visit are also applicable during the visit with the specialist. Presenting symptoms clearly and carefully is just as important when talking to a specialist. The same questions and suggestions we provided earlier can be used to guide you in your discussion. The physical examination also will be similar to what you receive from your primary-care physician; however, the examination will usually be limited to the area of the doctor's specialty.

There are a number of possible outcomes resulting from a visit to a specialist. These potential outcomes are listed below:

1. A diagnosis is reached and therapy is prescribed.
2. The specialist recommends surgery, either for diagnostic purposes or for therapeutic purposes.
3. A diagnosis cannot be made with the information obtained, and further testing is required.
4. The specialist refers you to another physician because a diagnosis still could not be made, and she feels you need to see someone with different expertise.
5. The specialist refers you back to the primary-care physician for monitoring of a physical finding or symptom.

Figure 19

Consultation Request

Dear _____ :

I am referring _____ to you for help with the following problem:

We have already obtained these studies:

It may help you to know that the patient also has these problems:

I would appreciate it if you would:
_____ Give me your opinion as to the diagnosis.
_____ Recommend management of the current problem.
_____ Assume full responsibility for management of this problem.
_____ Other _____

The patient is scheduled to return to see me _____

_____ M.D.   DATE: _____

Once an outcome has been reached, ask the specialist to discuss her recommendations. While you are in her office, get as much information from her as possible. Once again you can use the questions provided in earlier chapters to learn about your diagnosis, recommended testing, and planned treatment. This information will help you in making any necessary decisions and in discussing the results with your own doctor. It is also a good idea to ask the specialist how she will get back to your doctor to communicate results. This knowledge is particularly important to you and your doctor if the results indicate that additional procedures or treatments need to be done quickly.

Because you have already discussed with your primary-care doctor the possible tests and recommendations the specialist might make, her suggestions should sound familiar to you. If the specialist recommends an invasive procedure that you and your doctor have not discussed previously, make sure you talk to your doctor before agreeing to undergo the procedure. Similarly, if the specialist refers you to a third doctor, discuss the recommendation with your primary-care doctor before making the appointment.

Most of the time you will see the specialist for a short period of time and then be referred back to your primary-care doctor for follow-up. Occasionally you will continue to see the specialist for ongoing management of that problem. For example, a patient with severe arthritis may be followed chronically by a rheumatologist (a specialist in diseases of bones and joints) as various medications are tried. If this is the case, make sure there is continued communication between the specialist and your doctor. You can do this easily by asking the specialist to send to the primary-care doctor a copy of notes from each visit. As you can see, communication between you, your doctor, and the specialist is an extremely important facet of effective medical care.

12

Doctor-Patient Interactions

T hroughout this book, we have alluded to the importance of the patient-doctor relationship. This relationship is based on trust, confidence, and comfort; it facilitates professional as well as personal communication between you and your doctor. Although you may see your doctor only a few times a year, those minutes you spend together define the nature of your relationship. The factors that contribute to the success of this relationship go beyond the words exchanged and the information received. As with any type of communication, assumptions are made and feelings are affected throughout the course of the exchange. Misperceptions can occur, because patients or doctors may interpret the same information differently. The purpose of this chapter is to make you aware of the importance of interpersonal interactions between doctor and patient and of the impact they can have on your office visits.

Although we can help you prepare what to say and give you ways to secure information, we can't give you specific ways to prepare for the personal feelings and interactive style of you or your doctor. We've decided, therefore, that the most helpful way to bring your attention to these important areas would be to show you examples of positive and not-so-positive interactions. The scenarios are not designed to be teaching examples. We have not tried to provide answers—only explanations. In other words, the examples were not created to show how doctors or patients should or should not behave. They are, however, characteristic of how people *do* behave. The scenes were developed to provide some insight into how you or your doctor might interpret certain types of information or how either of you might perceive certain interactions. They are only possibilities.

Interaction

The first case is one of a forty-five-year-old carpenter who has had high blood pressure for three years. Initially he was reluctant to take medication, but once the decision was made for treatment, he has been very cooperative. He sees his doctor routinely for follow-up every three months.

Doctor: "How've you been? How's that new business doing?"

Patient: "Everything's going fine."

Doctor: "Any problems since the last time I saw you?"

Patient: "No, I'm doing fine."

Doctor: "Have you been taking your blood pressure medication daily?"

Patient: "Yes."

Doctor: "Any problems?"

Patient: "Well, it makes me a little drowsy, but I can live with it."

Doctor: "Do you want me to change the medication?"

Patient: "No, it really is no problem. I can live with it as long as my blood pressure is okay. I just wanted to let you know."

(After examination)

Doctor: "You're doing well. I'll see you again in three months."

Patient: "Do I need to continue taking the pills?"

Doctor: "Continue taking them and we'll see how you're doing in three months."

Reactions of the Doctor and Patient

The doctor likes seeing this patient.

The patient feels that the doctor really knows him on a personal level and is comfortable with the visit.

The interchange was one that fulfilled the doctor's "needs." The doctor felt good because the prescription worked and he felt the patient had been helped. The doctor also felt appreciative and pleased that the patient had been cooperative in taking medication as prescribed and that the patient was not afraid to be open and tell him about side effects.

The patient liked the fact that the doctor acknowledged the information he provided about the side effects. He was pleased that the doctor was willing to discuss changing medications because of his comments. The patient felt as if he had some control in his treatment.

Interpretation

In this dialogue, the interaction between the patient and doctor was a smooth one. It is important to a doctor to make a difference. When that desire is translated into day-to-day patient care, it means being able to do something of value and having the patient recognize the importance of the doctor's role in medical diagnosis and treatment. In this instance, the patient didn't actually have to say anything specific for his feelings of trust and confidence to come through.

Another important aspect of this dialogue is the implied level of comfort between the doctor and patient. A patient must feel the doctor really knows and cares about him before real comfort and ease can develop. This level of interaction is particularly important when, as in this situation, the patient has a chronic illness and will probably see the doctor on a fairly regular basis.

I n t e r a c t i o n

The second patient is a thirty-two-year-old secretary who noticed a breast lump two months ago. The doctor felt it was just a simple cyst but wanted to be certain. A mammogram was done and returned negative. Both the patient and the doctor know, however, that mammograms do not always detect breast tumors. The doctor does not think the lump feels suspicious enough to warrant a biopsy.

Doctor: "Hi. How have you been doing? Have you noticed any change in your breast since your last visit? Have you been checking it?"

Patient: "No, to be honest with you, it scares me and I haven't checked it at all."

Doctor: "I'm sorry to hear that you've been scared. I really don't think this is anything to worry about."

(After examination)

Doctor: "Well, I don't feel any change. If anything, it feels less significant. As we've discussed, your mammogram was normal. I think we can safely check it one more time in about three months, just to be certain."

Patient: "Are you sure there is nothing to worry about?"

Doctor: "No, I'm not positive—you can't be without a biopsy. But the likelihood of it being anything significant is exceedingly low."

Patient: "Well, what should we do?"

Doctor: "I'd prefer just to keep an eye on it for three months. If you'd feel more comfortable, we could always send you to a surgeon for a second opinion."

Patient: "What do you think?"

Doctor: "At this point I don't think you need to see a surgeon. We can just check it again in three months. If you do notice any change in your breast before then let me know, but I really don't think you have any cause for concern."

Patient: "Okay. I guess I'll see you again in three months."

Reactions of the Doctor and Patient

The doctor is comfortable with the decisions and with the physical signs indicating that the lump has become smaller.

The patient trusts the doctor's judgment and believes him. She is comfortable with the way he answers her questions.

The doctor feels he has presented the options and that the patient has agreed with his recommendation. He is pleased the patient seems to understand and accept that the lack of certainty in this situation is not a question of his ability but just the nature of the diagnostic process.

The patient believes the recommendations were based on sound medical judgment and not defensiveness, overconfidence, or arrogance. She is pleased that the doctor does not feel a biopsy is needed even though he can't give her a definitive answer without one.

The doctor is comfortable with his recommendation to wait yet realizes the consequences of that decision. He feels a very small degree of uncertainty until the next visit. Even though he thinks the lump is insignificant, the responsibility of the decision causes him some anxiety.

Although the patient feels relief about the doctor's recommendation, she also continues to have some anxiety because he wants to see her again in three months.

Interpretation

This dialogue revealed a patient and doctor who have developed a good interpersonal relationship. They are honest and open with each other. Yet the nature of the medical problem is such that it's impossible for either the doctor or the patient to end the visit completely satisfied and free from worry. The patient trusts the doctor's recommendation and has faith in his medical judgment. Even though she is not a suspicious person, she may be a little concerned that the doctor wants to bring her in to check the lump again in three months. Perhaps she fears that the doctor is not telling her all of the possibilities because they are unlikely and he doesn't want to worry her. On the other hand, the doctor believes he is keeping her from receiving unnecessary surgery. Yet he feels very acutely the responsibility of his decision that the lump is not significant. Even though he is almost positive of this, he wants another opportunity to confirm his diagnosis, even though it may cause the patient a little further worry.

Interaction

The third patient is a sixty-two-year-old woman with a history of treatment for high blood pressure and arthritis. She has been seeing this doctor regularly for six years. Last year she was hospitalized with pneumonia but has been doing quite well since then.

Doctor: "How have you been doing?"

Patient: "I'm not doing well at all."

Doctor: "I'm sorry to hear that. What's the matter?"

Patient: "When I stand up I feel like I'm going to pass out."

Doctor: "How long has this been going on?"

Patient: "About two weeks and my feet are hurting me, too. I think it's my arthritis again."

Doctor: "Let's not worry about your feet right now. Tell me more about the lightheadedness. Does it happen only when you stand? How long does it last?"

Patient: "Yes, it happens when I stand up. It gets better in a few minutes when I sit back down."

(After examination)

Doctor: "Mrs. Jackson, I think your blood pressure drops too low when you stand up. That is the reason you feel lightheaded. We'll have to adjust your medication to keep that from happening."

Patient: "Okay. But what should we do about my feet?"

Doctor: "We'll deal with that when I see you next—I think your next appointment is in six weeks."

Reactions of the Doctor and Patient

The doctor feels happy that she made a quick diagnosis of a potentially serious problem. She knows that if the foot problem is anything significant, she will be able to check it out the next time she sees Mrs. Jackson—when she is less busy. She is confident about the overall success of the visit.

The patient feels the doctor ignored her foot problem. That fact has preoccupied her during her visit. She thinks the doctor was supposed to address all of the problems she presented and is concerned that the doctor didn't take her complaint seriously.

The doctor considered the patient's problems and solved the most significant one. She is not particularly concerned about the foot problem mentioned. The quality of the interaction doesn't even cross her mind. She would be very surprised to know that the visit disturbed the patient in any way.

The patient is generalizing her concern over this problem to her overall evaluation of the doctor's behavior. She begins to think that the doctor doesn't act as if she has time for her anymore. She thinks maybe it is time to change doctors.

Although the doctor and the patient have heard the same words, the interpretations have been quite different. The doctor wouldn't have a clue that the patient was even considering leaving her for another doctor.

Interpretation

In this situation, the doctor is satisfied and the patient is not. The doctor addressed her priority concern—the woman's dizziness—and identified the source of the problem. She was able to eliminate the major issue and the only one that could have been potentially dangerous or life threatening. The patient may have been unaware of the doctor's priority or that her fainting symptom was a real cause for concern. The patient's major concern was her arthritic pain, which she was having to deal with on a day-to-day basis. The doctor didn't focus at all on this particular problem. Although the patient presented only two problems, the doctor didn't attend to the symptom of foot pain. It may have been that the doctor spent more time on the first problem than she expected, or it may be that she simply didn't pay enough attention to a complaint she had heard many times before. This lack of attention to what was a major area of concern to the patient and a minor area of concern to the doctor led to a significant sense of dissatisfaction on the part of the patient. The doctor did not recognize the potential for the patient's unhappiness because she didn't recognize the importance of the symptom to the patient.

Interaction

The fourth patient is a thirty-seven-year-old accountant who has seen the doctor only twice in the last three years—once for a routine exam, the other time for a sore throat. He had an appointment for a visit later next week but asked to be worked in today because of his concern about recent chest pains.

Doctor: "Bill, you're a week early for your appointment. What's the problem?"

Patient: "I've been having chest pains lately. I've been a little worried about them."

Doctor: "How often have they been occurring?"

Patient: "About once a week."

Doctor: "Where in your chest is the pain?"

(Patient points to the left side of his chest)

Doctor: "How long does the pain last?"

Patient: "Just a few seconds. It feels like a stab."

Doctor: "Does it ever last longer?"

Patient: "No."
Doctor: "When does it come?"
Patient: "When I'm sitting at my desk."
Doctor: "Has it come when you exercise?"
Patient: "No."

(After examination)

Doctor: "Bill, your chest pain is not serious. It's probably just a muscle spasm."
Patient: "How do you know it's not my heart?"
Doctor: "Because your pain only lasts for a few seconds, is sharp, and never comes on with exertion. Heart pain usually lasts longer, feels like tightening, and typically comes on with exercise."
Patient: "Don't you think I need a stress test to be sure it's not my heart? Should I see a specialist?"
Doctor: "No, I don't think it's necessary."
Patient: "Well, then, how can you be sure it's not heart pain?"
Doctor: "Because what you've described to me is not heart pain, for the reasons I've already mentioned."

Reactions of the Doctor and Patient

The doctor is certain the patient does not have heart disease. She is irritated that the patient persists in questioning her diagnosis despite her good explanation.

The patient wants to know why the doctor won't order a stress test. He questions the doctor's conclusion without a test.

The doctor feels she has been very thorough. She feels she has saved the patient unnecessary tests and expense and is a little upset because it appears the patient places more value in the test than in her clinical judgment.

The patient is concerned and is not convinced the diagnosis is correct. He considers making an appointment with a specialist to get a "more complete" examination.

The doctor realizes the patient is dissatisfied, but her own resentment and the knowledge that the diagnosis is correct override her concern about the patient's feelings and possible reactions.

Interpretation

At the conclusion of the above dialogue, the patient is still unsure of the diagnosis and may go to see another doctor. The doctor is irritated and somewhat offended by the exchange. The basic issue is that the patient was scared by the pains that he felt. He wanted to be absolutely certain he was not experiencing signs of a heart condition. The patient considered his questions about a stress test and a specialist perfectly logical and justified in this situation. He certainly wasn't thinking of the possibility that the doctor would be upset by his requests for reassurance. The doctor's reaction to this and similar situations may stem from a generalized reaction to patients who seem to question repeatedly her diagnostic ability. Although patients often are looking for confirmation or evidence of a diagnosis, the doctor may sometimes feel as if her skill or ability is being overlooked as the patient asks repeatedly for other tests or the opinion of a specialist. This is more likely to be the case when the diagnosis is very obvious and clear-cut to the physician. As with any individual who has pride in her skills, the doctor may unfortunately get a little defensive when those skills are inadvertently or consciously questioned.

Interaction

The fifth patient is a forty-five-year-old plant supervisor with chronic high blood pressure. He has seen the doctor for three years for routine follow-up visits. Both his wife and son are also patients of this doctor.

Doctor: "Hey, Jim, how are you doing?"

Patient: "Well, my blood pressure was okay last week when I had it checked by the nurse at work. But I'm sure it's high now after spending an hour in your waiting room."

Doctor: "Don't give me a hard time, Jim. I was in the emergency room until midnight and I'm not in the mood to argue. Just take your shirt off and I'll be back in a minute to examine you. By the way, are you having any problems?"

Patient: "Well, I guess not." (Jim has experienced some abdominal pain recently, but after this exchange he doesn't feel comfortable mentioning it.)

Doctor: "Are you sure?"

Patient: "Yes."

(After examination)

Doctor: "Your blood pressure is normal. Stay on the same medication and I'll see you again in about three months."

R e a c t i o n s   o f   t h e   D o c t o r   a n d   P a t i e n t

The patient is angry about the wait. He still feels it was the doctor's fault that he was out there for an hour but then felt embarrassed after the doctor's comments. He's upset with the way the doctor spoke to him.

The doctor is angry at the way the patient voiced his complaint. He feels ashamed of himself, however, for getting angry and defensive. He feels his patient just doesn't understand how hard he works.

The patient feels humiliated, as if the doctor has chastised him. He just wants to get out of the office and doesn't mention the fact that he has experienced some pain in his stomach.

The doctor feels disturbed that the patient showed irritation at the wait, particularly because they previously had a good relationship.

The patient leaves wondering how he will feel the next time he comes to see this doctor. He feels uncomfortable about the visit, and isn't sure if he should call the doctor and make another appointment about his stomach pain.

The doctor tries to suppress his feelings of anger and hopes they don't carry over to his next patient.

Interpretation

In this scene, we have seen how an issue that is related neither to the patient's medical condition nor the doctor's medical skill can cause serious damage to the patient-doctor relationship. The patient was upset that he had to wait an hour for his appointment. Because he was angry, he presented his legitimate complaint in an inflammatory manner. The doctor responded accordingly, and the rest of the exchange was tense and uncomfortable. Both the patient and the doctor were reacting not only to what was said but also to their perceptions of what the other was thinking or feeling. For example, the patient might have felt the wait was due to the doctor's arrogance and lack of respect for the patient's time. The doctor may have felt the patient didn't understand how hard he had been working during the last twenty-four hours. If the patient's comment had been less provocative, or if the doctor had been able to respond calmly, the visit might have ended on a more pleasant note. The biggest problem with this type of interaction is that the assessment or treatment of the patient's medical problem may be compromised. This may happen because time and attention are focused on nonmedical issues or, as in this case, because the patient didn't want to prolong the visit.

S u m m a r y

In earlier discussions we've illustrated different parts of the diagnostic process. In this chapter we have shown you typical examples of the interactions between doctors and their patients. There is no definite right or wrong in most of these dialogues, although you might have felt differently when you read them. As you've read this chapter, we hope you have noticed the importance of mutual respect and open communication. It may have appeared more evident in those interactions that seemed most effective. You also have had a chance to look at the logic or the train of thought followed by the doctor when he makes a decision related to testing or treatment. By providing you with "behind-the-scenes" information related to interpersonal relationships, we hope we have provided you with a glimpse of some possible rationales, perceptions, and concerns that you or your doctor might have. We have tried to use the text in this chapter as another way to bridge the gap of understanding between the physician and patient and how each sees the other.

13

Tips for Patients

How to Minimize Waiting

Waiting in a doctor's office has become an expected inconvenience. Sometimes it's justified, sometimes it isn't. Our purpose is not to review the reasons for waiting. Instead, we want to help you solve the problem.

The best time to schedule a routine follow-up visit is the first appointment after your doctor's lunch hour. The next-best time is the first appointment in the morning. The former is better because lunch is a less likely source of delay than hospitalized patients, whom the doctor will see in the morning. If there are no other patients scheduled before you, you will be the first one seen unless an extremely ill patient comes in unexpectedly.

If you call and ask to be seen the day of your call or in the next day or two, you should assume that your doctor's schedule is full and that he will have to work you into it. Unless you are very ill, you should expect a wait in this type of situation. Ask the nurse what time would most likely result in the least waiting time. Ask about the time right after lunch; there always is the possibility that it will be open. If not, ask if any patients have cancelled and if you could fill that slot. If you must schedule in the middle of the afternoon, realize that it is the worst time to work in unscheduled patients. It is unfair to have the smooth schedule of all the other patients disrupted to minimize your wait. You should ask how long your wait might be if you must come in at that time. An additional tip: it can lessen a lot of your frustration, as those minutes tick by, if you bring a book you really want to read. Don't rely on the doctor's magazines. It's better to become engrossed in a good novel than in how slowly the minute hand moves.

How to Convey Your Complaints to Your Doctor

You have a right to let your doctor know if there is something wrong, but do it at the right time—the end of the office visit. When you start out with a complaint, you are guaranteed to get your doctor thinking about how to defend herself instead of thinking about the medical problem that brought you there in the first place. After everything is completed—the interview, the exam, the doctor's explanation—bring the issue up with your doctor. Don't be timid. Let the doctor know if there's a problem, but seek a solution, not a confrontation. Statements such as "Doctor, I had to wait an hour to be seen today. What's the best time to schedule an office visit to minimize waiting?" are more likely to get you a satisfactory response.

How to Inform Your Doctor About Problems with the Staff

The doctor is not the only one you will see in the office. You will spend a lot of time with nurses and office staff. It

is important for you to get along well with them as well
as with your doctor. Otherwise, you will feel less comfortable in his office and may even hesitate to call when
needed because you "don't want to deal with the nurse up
front." Never assume that your doctor knows how all of
the staff members treat the patients. As with any other
complaint, mention it to the doctor at the end of the office
visit. Remember to judge the staff from their typical behavior rather than from one incident.

How to Phrase Phone Requests

If your problem is a true emergency, something that you
think could require hospitalization, you or whoever calls
for you should ask the nurse to interrupt the doctor instead of requesting a call back. A slip of paper stating
"Mrs. Smith says to call her back immediately" could possibly end up on the doctor's desk underneath another patient's request for a prescription refill. In such a situation,
do not take no or "The doctor will call you back when she
can" as an answer. On the other hand, a doctor should
not be interrupted unless it is a true emergency. It is unfair to the patient she is seeing in the office at the time of
your call.

If you have a medical problem, call as early in the day
as possible. If you wait until late in the day, the doctor's
office could close and she might have to see you in the
emergency room. This would be much less desirable and
much more expensive for you. If you think your problem
is something that could require a visit to the office, you
should let the receptionist know that when you call. It is
very likely that the doctor will call back earlier because
she will have to decide when to work you into the schedule. Also, most doctors want to have an idea of how many

patients they will be seeing during the day. Keep the phone line open. Otherwise, the doctor may call when she has a spare moment, get a busy signal, and not have another chance to try for an hour or two. On the other hand, if you think it's likely she will need to see you, it's almost always best just to go ahead and schedule an appointment rather than first waiting several hours for a call and having to come in anyway.

Sometimes it may be difficult for you to judge whether or not you need to come in to see the doctor before you've had a chance to speak to her. If your problem involves something that needs to be looked at in order for the doctor to give an opinion (a new mole, a swollen foot), definitely set up an appointment. If you're calling because you think you may need an antibiotic, it also is usually best to schedule a visit. Most doctors do not like to prescribe antibiotics for new problems over the telephone. If, however, your question is about a possible side effect of a medicine or the worsening of a chronic problem, you may be able to get an adequate answer with just a call. When you are calling for the results of a test or with a question that clearly would not require an office visit (i.e., how long to take a medicine), it is quite possible that the nurse could answer the question after first discussing it with the doctor. If there still is something you need to talk about with the doctor (i.e., what to do about an elevated blood-cholesterol count), ask the nurse to have her call you after her last patient. Find out when that will be so you don't need to sit at home all day waiting for a call. Instead, you can return around the time the doctor will call you.

Calling for Prescription Refills

Again, call as early as possible for prescription refills. Avoid calling for refills after office hours or on weekends.

If you call during those times, your doctor won't have your chart with him so he won't be able to double-check the accuracy of the prescription. It is also possible that you may get your doctor's associate, who won't know your medication at all.

Never call for a refill from the pharmacy. If you go there first, you may have a long wait before the doctor can be interrupted to confirm your prescription. Call from home or work and ask the receptionist approximately when the prescription will be phoned in to the pharmacy. Always give the telephone number of your pharmacy to the receptionist who takes your call. Otherwise, you will have to wait until the receptionist has the time to find the number before your request even gets to the doctor.

What Records to Transfer When You Change Doctors

Moving to another city has become common in our mobile society. You will want your new doctor to know the details of your medical history. A knowledge of past test results could influence her decisions should you become ill in the future. As soon as you realize you are moving, ask your doctor to copy the records we list below. Give as much advance notice as possible; copying records is probably the lowest priority in a doctor's office. Copies of records to request include:

- most recent complete physical exam
- records from hospitalizations
- all specialists' consultations
- most recent X-ray reports
- most recent EKG
- most recent lab studies (e.g., blood and urine tests)
- office notes detailing any significant illnesses

Most doctors will not give you the original records for medical-legal reasons. Some doctors do not charge for copying records, but don't be surprised if there is a small fee.

How to Decrease the Amount You Spend on Medicines

There are several ways to lower your medication costs significantly. Brand-name drugs are nearly always more expensive than generic drugs (same drugs, different names). In most cases, the generic drug is equally effective. You will frequently save money if you ask your doctor to prescribe generic substitutions. Realize, however, there are several exceptions in which the brand-name drug is superior because the generic equivalent does not get adequately absorbed into the body. Most doctors are familiar with these exceptions. You should ask both your doctor and your pharmacist if the generic substitute prescribed is as effective as the brand-name medication.

Always let your doctor know if the cost of your medication is a significant concern. There may be a less expensive alternative. This is particularly true with blood-pressure pills and antibiotics. Your doctor may not always be aware of price differences, however, so you might also ask your pharmacist. Before filling your prescription, you can call several pharmacies for price quotes. The differences can be considerable, particularly for expensive medications. Also, one drugstore may be cheaper for one medication than for another, so you might use more than one pharmacy if you take several medications. If you do this, however, make sure each pharmacy knows all the medicines you take, so each can monitor for drug interactions.

A less obvious way to save money is to ask your doctor

or your pharmacist if the medication comes in a pill form that can be broken in half. It can sometimes be much less expensive to get a dosage twice as strong and take half the pill. For example, instead of taking a 100-milligram pill twice a day, you could take half of a 200-milligram pill twice a day.

Conclusion

In this book we have discussed the importance of having a competent primary-care physician and your role in the diagnostic process. In the first four chapters we have explored the ways to identify and select a good doctor. As you've seen, there are many skills a good doctor must possess. Now that you have become more aware of these, you know how to look for them in your present doctor or when you go to select a new one.

The last nine chapters have given you the information you need to participate more fully in the diagnostic and treatment process. Your next visit to your doctor's office should be less stressful and more comfortable. You now have a good idea of what is happening while you are there, and why. You should be more prepared to give accurate and concise information, understand how your doctor makes a diagnosis, and feel more confident talking to him about his conclusions. We hope you use the information provided in this book and use it consistently. It will make a difference—to you and to your doctor.

Glossary of Major Medical and Surgical Specialists

Medical Specialists

Allergist. Diagnoses and treats conditions causing unusual sensitivity to different substances, such as pollens, dusts, and insect stings. Typical reasons for referral include frequent sinus infections, allergic asthma, and severe reactions to bee stings.

Cardiologist. Diagnoses and treats diseases of the heart and blood vessels. Reasons for referral include an abnormal heartbeat, evaluation of chest pain, and heart attack.

Dermatologist. Diagnoses and treats diseases of the skin, hair, and nails. Reasons for referral include rashes, hair loss, and an abnormal mole.

Endocrinologist. Diagnoses and treats abnormalities of the hormone-secreting glands such as the thyroid, pancreas, ovaries, and gonads. Typical reasons for referral include poorly controlled diabetes, early menopause, and an overactive thyroid gland.

Gastroenterologist. Diagnoses and treats diseases of the organs of the digestive system such as the esophagus, stomach, intestines, and liver. Reasons for referral include ulcers, hepatitis, and colon polyps.

Hematologist. Diagnoses and treats diseases of the blood. Reasons for referral include anemia, leukemia, and abnormal bleeding.

Nephrologist. Diagnoses and treats diseases of the kidneys. Reasons for referral include abnormal function of the kidneys and kidney failure requiring dialysis.

Neurologist. Diagnoses and treats diseases of the nervous system. Reasons for referral include seizures, unusual headaches, and strokes.

Obstetrician-Gynecologist (OBGYN). Diagnoses and treats abnormalities of the female reproductive system and delivers babies. Reasons for referral include abnormal vaginal bleeding, enlarged ovary, and pregnancy. This specialist also performs surgery on the uterus and ovaries.

Oncologist. Diagnoses and treats cancer. Reasons for referral include medical management of various cancers, such as colon, lung, or breast.

Psychiatrist. Diagnoses and treats mental disorders. Reasons for referral include severe depression, extreme anxiety, and eating disorders.

Pulmonologist. Diagnoses and treats diseases of the lung. Reasons for referral include coughing up blood, emphysema, and an abnormal chest X ray.

Rheumatologist. Diagnoses and medically treats diseases of the bones, joints, and muscles. Reasons for referral include arthritis, gout, and lupus.

Surgical Specialists

Cardiovascular surgeon. Specializes in the surgical treatment of diseases of the heart and blood vessels. Reasons for referral include open-heart surgery, aneurysm repair, and mending a torn blood vessel (for example, from a bullet wound).

General surgeon. Surgically treats a variety of diseases.

Typical reasons for referral include gallstones, appendicitis, and hernias.

Neurosurgeon. Specializes in the surgical treatment of abnormalities of the brain and spinal cord. Reasons for referral include removal of a brain tumor and operations on the spinal cord.

Ophthalmologist. Diagnoses diseases of the eye and performs surgery when necessary. Reasons for referral include glaucoma, decreasing vision, and cataract removal.

Orthopedic surgeon. Specializes in the surgical treatment of abnormalities of the spine, bones, and joints. Reasons for referral include severe back pain, fractures, and shoulder injuries.

Otolaryngologist (ENT). Specializes in the diagnosis and surgical treatment of diseases involving the ears, nose, and throat. Reasons for referral include deafness, nosebleeds, and persistent hoarseness.

Plastic surgeon. Specializes in cosmetic surgery and correction of disfiguring injuries. Reasons for referral include breast augmentation, scar removal, and skin grafting.

Proctologist. Specializes in the surgical treatment of problems of the colon and rectum. Reasons for referral include hemorrhoid repair and surgical removal of colon cancer.

Urologist. Specializes in the diagnosis and surgical treatment of diseases of the kidney, bladder, and prostate. Reasons for referral include kidney stones, prostate enlargement, and impotence.

Index